Eating Between the Lines

Eating Between the Lines

THE SUPERMARKET SHOPPER'S GUIDE
TO THE TRUTH BEHIND FOOD LABELS

KIMBERLY LORD STEWART

St. Martin's Griffin ⚑ New York

American Grassfed logo courtesy of American Grassfed Association, Denver, Colorado, www.americangrassfed.org; American Humane Association Free Farm Certified logo courtesy of American Humane Association, Denver, Colorado, www.americanhumane.org; American Lamb logo courtesy of American Lamb Board, Denver, Colorado, www.americanlambboard.org; Best Aquaculture Practices Certified logo courtesy of Aquaculture Certification Alliance, Kirkland, Washington, www.aquaculture certification.org; Bird Friendly logo courtesy of Smithsonian Migratory Bird Center, National Zoological Park, Washington, D.C., www.nationalzoo.si.edu; California Olive Oil Council logo courtesy of California Olive Oil Council, Berkeley, California, www.cooc.org; cartoon image of grapes being washed, Safe Handling Instructions card, Thermy cartoon, and irradiation symbol courtesy of the Food Safety and Inspection Service; Certified Humane, Raised and Handled logo courtesy of Certified Humane, Raised and Handled, Herndon, Virginia, www.certifiedhumane.org; Certified Naturally Grown logo courtesy of Certified Naturally Grown, New Paltz, New York, www.naturallygrown.org; Chianti Classico logo courtesy of Consorzio Del Marchio Storico, Chianti Classico, San Casciano, Italy, www.chianticlas sico.com; Coffee Kids logo courtesy of Coffee Kids, Santa Fe, New Mexico, www.coffeekids.org; Colorado Proud logo courtesy of Colorado Proud, Colorado State Department of Agriculture, www.ag.state .co.us; Demeter Certified Biodynamic logo courtesy of the Demeter Association, Inc., Philomath, Oregon, www.demeter-usa.org; Dolphin Safe symbol courtesy of the U.S. Department of Commerce; Fair Trade logo courtesy of Trans Fair USA, Oakland, California, www.transfairusa.org; Fresh Q Label logo courtesy of Food Quality Sensor International, www.fqsinternational.com; Health Claims report card courtesy of FDA; Homeland Security Advisory System image courtesy of the Department of Homeland Security; IPM symbol courtesy of IPM Institute of North America; Kona Coffee logo courtesy of Kona Coffee Farmers Association, Kailua-Kona, Hawaii, www.konacoffeefarmers.org; kosher symbols courtesy of Union of Orthodox Jewish Congregations, the Organized Kashrus Laboratories, Star-K Kosher Certification, and KOF-K Kosher Certification; Live and Active Cultures logo courtesy of National Yogurt Association, McLean, Virginia, www.aboutyogurt.com; Low Glycemic logos courtesy of Glycemic Institute, Washington, D.C., www.glycemic.com; Marine Stewardship Council logo courtesy of Marine Stewardship Council, London, England, www.msc.org; National Wildlife Federation logo courtesy of National Wildlife Federation, Reston, Virginia, www.nwf.org; NSF logo courtesy of NSF International, Ann Arbor, Michigan, www.nsf.org; Protected Harvest logo courtesy of Protected Harvest, San Diego, California, Randy Duckworth, executive director of the Wisconsin Potato & Vegetable Growers Association, www.protectedharvest.org; Rainforest Alliance Certified logo courtesy of the Rainforest Alliance, New York, www.rainforest-alliance.com; REAL logo courtesy of Dairy Management, Inc., Rosemont, Illinois, www.dairyinfo.com; Safe Harbor Certified Seafood logo courtesy of Seafood Safe, LLC, Dover, (continued on page 314)

www.stmartins.com

Library of Congress Cataloging-in-Publication Data
Stewart, Kimberly Lord.
    Eating between the lines: the supermarket shopper's guide to the truth behind food labels / Kimberly Lord Stewart.
        p.   cm.
    ISBN-13: 978-0-312-34774-1
    ISBN-10: 0-312-34774-X
    1. Food—Labeling.   I. Title
TP374.5.S74 2007
613.2—dc22   2006051015

10   9   8   7   6   5   4   3

To my Round Table Knights and Dames,
the Archers, Lords, and Stewarts

Due to increasing knowledge and consumer interest, food ingredients, label practices, and regulatory requirements are changing regularly. It is possible that some things in this book may have changed by the time you read it. Likewise, Internet Web sites may have changed or disappeared between when this book was written and when it is read. Further, the fact that an organization or Web site is referred to as a citation and/or potential source of further information does not mean that the author or the publisher endorses the information the organization or Web site may provide or recommendations it may make.

CONTENTS

ACKNOWLEDGMENTS

When I started writing this book and told others about it, the most frequent question was—are you writing about the entire grocery store? The answer, yes, may question my good sense, as there are more than 40,000 products in the average grocery store. I couldn't possibly address every label and expect to publish a book before dementia set in, so I've tried to cover topics that occupy most food shoppers' minds, such as health messages, food-production issues like organic farming and pesticide and antibiotics use, as well as animal-welfare claims.

It seems like a lot of information to digest, but in reality, if your pantry and refrigerator were completely bare and you needed to fill them in one shopping trip, this book would encapsulate every thought, question, and subliminal decision-making process you might have while grocery shopping. My best advice to shoppers is to remember that when trying to interpret food labels and marketing claims, it's not about how well educated one is—after all, they are written for consumers, not physicians, nutritionists, or food scientists.

While the complexity behind the decision-making process may require a postgraduate education, food labels are supposed to be targeted for the likes of you and me—the average shopper. Like on a string attached to two cans, somewhere amid the lines of communication between very brilliant scientists and eager shoppers trying to make the right choices, the messages lose clarity. If anything, I am a conduit who tries to connect the tin cans on either end and not let the interference in the middle drown out the message.

Often shoppers interpret food labels to mean what they hope or think they mean—not necessarily what is so. If I have any particular advantage over the average person standing in line with me in the grocery store, it is that I spend a lot of time talking with and reading research done by very intelligent people who grow our food, raise the livestock, milk the cows, fish the seas, and communicate the health and science of the four basic foods groups.

There are too many to mention here, but all too often these behind-the-scenes experts in the fields, farms, and laboratories don't get the credit they deserve. Consider this heartfelt gratitude for all you have done for me. What's more, I couldn't have taken on such a large project without the help of fellow journalists, the staff editors at *Natural Foods Merchandiser* magazine, my former employer and a trade publication for the health-food industry, and the journalists at *Food Navigator*. Both fill my e-mail in-box daily with news and insights about the inner workings of the food world, and while they are a hefty read for consumers, if you really want to know more about your food, sign up for their newsletters at www.foodnavigator.com and www.newhope.com. In addition, I thank the journalists with the Food Safety and Inspection Service at the U.S. Department of Agriculture for their clear and concise work, well done.

On more than one occasion while writing this book, I've stood in a grocery store aisle furiously scribbling notes or asking too many questions—I appreciate the tolerance shown by the clerks at the King Soopers grocery store in Longmont, Colorado. I'm equally grateful to the Colorado farmers who never fail to offer a smile and answer my questions when I ride in on my blue bike to the farmers' market on Saturdays, even though they've spent the previous week working through droughts, heat waves, as well as late-spring and early-fall snows to provide the best food Colorado soil can offer.

To my agent, Judith Weber, my editor, Michael Flamini, and his editorial assistant, Vicki Lame, at St. Martin's Press, your trust in me that I could take on such a big and dynamic first project as this one is astonishing. At times it was daunting, but your patience and kind support were encouraging.

A gazillion thanks to my family, who put up with my long hours and tired mind during the many months of writing. Finally, there aren't enough words in any dictionary to express appreciation to my husband, who transitioned gracefully and exceptionally from flying U.S. Navy jets to being a scribe's finest editor.

Playing with Our Minds and Our Food

The idea for this book came about in the olive oil section of my local grocery store. I had just won a journalism award for an article in *The Denver Post* about some slippery tactics in the olive oil industry regarding fraudulent labeling and adulteration. I was in the baking aisle, picking out my usual brand of Italian olive oil, when I noticed a woman holding a bottle of oil in each hand. With her eyeglasses perched on the bridge of her nose, she carefully studied the labels. I moved on, but passed by the same aisle ten minutes later—she was still there.

I felt her pain. "I know a little bit about this; can I help you?" I asked. Without any hesitation or worry that I might be a purse snatcher, she admitted defeat and handed me the bottles. I walked her through the ins and outs of olive oil labeling, and by the end of our conversation she said, "Can you go shopping with me all the time?" That isn't the best use of my time, but it was a good idea for a book.

My food knowledge comes from a broad range of people and professions. First, as a parent, I care about what my kids eat. As they get older, I have about as much control of their eating habits as I do their taste in music. But I see spoonfuls of hope when my college-age son calls to say he's inviting friends over for Sunday dinner and asks how to stuff a pork roast, or when my high school son tells his friends about trans fat in their junk food.

I took the long way around to becoming a journalist and food writer. My interest in food began while working as a Pan Am flight attendant. I was nineteen years old and the world was my table. The rest of my family lived in Germany, while my father, who raised me, was the U.S. Air Force attaché at the embassy and my mother an international fashion model. When home, I wined and dined with heads of state. It was the height of the Cold War, and the mood was very cloak-and-dagger. The food and spirits were equally intriguing—one evening might be spent with my father and his cronies drinking Arctic-cold vodka with the Russians; the next night my dad would coax me to eat jellyfish salad with the South Korean ambassador.

As a flight attendant, I learned to cook in a first-class cabin, hanging 35,000 feet in the air. On layovers, I experienced lamb curry with a brass merchant's family in India. I learned the elegant art of Japanese tea ceremonies and how to gracefully fend off advances from male tea-shop owners. I celebrated my twenty-first birthday on the island of Fiji with fellow crew members, tropical drinks, and a fresh banana cake. I sat elbow to elbow with sweaty beer-drinking expatriates in Liberia, while we muscled each other for just caught, steamed prawns, prepared by a charming Belgian chef (very surreal . . .).

My mother fueled my interest in food at an early age. She is an elegant hostess with a keen awareness in health and fitness—a Mother Earth in Prada. Whether she was playing tennis, gliding down the catwalks at European fashion houses as a model, or chasing my younger siblings, few people knew about her pain and discomfort from a lifelong autoimmune disease, lupus. After years of misdiagnoses and surviving cancer, she traded in her drugs for a new diet and a vitamin regimen. Naturally, it was a family project. We had not eaten poorly before, but this new diet emphasized the importance of vitamin C–packed foods, wheat germ (it showed up on our morning cereal and in chocolate-chip cookies), as well as locally sourced milk and eggs from small farms. Today I, too, show signs of the disease, so I am grateful for all she taught me.

When I became a U.S. Navy wife, my jet-jockey husband and I settled into domesticity. In between too many six to eight month–long deployments, we had two boys, moved to a house tucked into a hundred-acre walnut orchard, and I started a catering business. With one boy in a playpen, the other in a backpack, I cooked for residents in the tiny town of Hanford, California (population 6,000). I got to know California's farm-belt natives and the peach, walnut, almond, tomato, and cotton crops that sustain them. Our budget was tighter than the collar on my husband's dress-white uniform, so I dabbled in farming and canning with the encouragement of my farmer father, whom I had been estranged from since a young age. He counseled me on when to plant and how to tend the fruit trees, and I discovered the best way to restore a long-damaged relationship—one season at a time.

Later the navy shipped us to a tiny village in Italy called Gaeta. My weekly shopping at the market on the piazza was a lesson in the value of local foods and how a relationship with farmers is vital to the strength of the economy and the health of the community. The village was a middle-class fishing and shipping port about an hour south of Rome. Each evening the fishermen set up tables along the *lunga mare,* the promenade by the sea, to sell their daily catch. The freshest fish I'd ever seen, with names I still can't remember, lay blanketed in crushed ice.

What impressed me most was the tolerance among the grocers and local farmers. My produce lady, Yolanda, and her teenage sons set up their stand every morning directly in front of the grocery store, with no questions asked. The store manager unlocked the front door each morning, waved to Yolanda, and got on with his day. Each Wednesday the same market square was filled with even more pro-duce sellers, bakers, olive and deli carts, pasta makers, florists, and shoe vendors. There was no bickering as to which food was better tasting or better for you. Each merchant lived in harmony with the others, under a symbiotic understanding that none could survive with-out the customer traffic each merchant attracted.

The first time I ventured down the hill to shop at Yolanda's, my rookie status was evident. My Italian was poor; at the time I could buy the essentials: shoes, cappuccino, and pizza. Yolanda was a little scary; her fingers were bent and permanently lined with dirt from pulling vegetables that grew sweet in the red Italian soil. It was her bark that unnerved me the most. Each time she saw me coming down the hill, she bayed in a deep, dusty voice. As my Italian improved, I recognized she was advertising, not her shop—but me. "The *Americana*!

The *Americana* shops here. Come! Come and buy!" she shouted. I reveled in my celebrity status. She never failed to fill my basket with more than I paid for and more than I could carry back up the steep cobblestone hill.

By the time I moved to Colorado in 1994, I was ready to finish what I had put off for too long, a college degree. My intent was to be a nutritionist; however, my wanderlust and curiosity were too strong for a clinical career. I found the perfect fit with journalism and an emphasis in food and health.

My first job was as an editorial intern for New Hope Natural Media. At my age—well into my thirties—I needed experience fast. Foolish, but I offered to work for free for six months, doing anything required to gain enough experience to find a paying job. At the end of the internship, I was hired on full-time. For the next five years, I worked my way from an intern to executive editor of *Natural Food Merchandiser,* the leading trade magazine for the health-food industry, and director of Internet content for a related trade and consumer Web site.

During my tenure, the once poor entrepreneurs who started their health-food businesses while sleeping in VW buses became the new millionaires. Suddenly this hippie-food fad was mainstream. Health food was king for conventional groceries interested in improving the bottom line. Moreover, marketers had a fresh dictionary of buzzwords, like "free-range," "hormone-free," "organic," and "natural." As a journalist, I was fascinated with the new lingo. From a consumer vantage point it was often confusing, deceptive, and ridiculous, which is where the seed for *Eating Between the Lines* grew into a full-fledged book.

In America, I miss Yolanda's daily produce selection and her pull-no-punches marketing. Unfortunately, in this country, the food industry communicates with customers through food labels, marketing, and advertising more than relationships. Every time you walk through those big double doors you are faced with as many as 40,000 different products. And just when you think you know them all, a new one comes along. No wonder we never stick to our shopping lists.

The impulse to buy is too tempting, and with all those marketing messages and labels screaming at us, it's hard not to get distracted. My family has been known to send out a search party for me in the grocery store—they know, when I say we just need a few things, I'll be gone for a while. As a food journalist, though, I'm not one to latch on to every magic-bullet product that comes along. It took some time for me to be convinced that sometimes the least expensive foods are not always the best choice, other times the bargain is worth it.

Perhaps no other American product has as much competition as food. One might think with our aging demographic and slowing population growth, the number of new products in the store would level off. Not so; publicly traded corporations that answer to the bottom line have but one mantra—sell, sell, sell. Since we all eat at least three times a day, we need food, but the habit of buying and eating *more* than we need is contributing to not only wastefulness but also *waistfulness*.

Eating Between the Lines is an explanation of all the tactics—legal, ethical, and otherwise—that food companies use to get us to buy their product and, better yet, buy it again. Beyond avoiding starvation and hunger, the reasons we buy one food brand over another are complicated. It's a matter of taste preference, brand loyalty, price, convenience, health, and even social values.

Unlike the majority of the world's poorer populations, who worry about getting enough to eat, we have esoteric choices of *want* rather than need. Whittle away the nonessential aspects of eating, such as pleasure and entertainment, the real reason we eat is to stay alive, but the overabundance of products alters our perception of food to a lifestyle choice, rather than life support.

Behind each of our decisions for one brand or one type of food over another is a food-marketing expert designing products, advertising, and labels to get our attention and make their product—which is rubbing labels with hundreds of other products—practically jump into the cart. Depending on the message, labels trigger our buying decisions. And, because food shopping is no longer as much about a lasting relationship with the butcher or the produce farmer, we rely on labels as a source of trustworthy information. But not all labels on products are verified by a private third-party or government agency, leaving manufacturers with a lot of freedom to say whatever they think will motivate a shopper to buy and leaving the consumer wondering what is fact or fiction.

Right now the only way for anyone to understand all the labels in the grocery store is to call the manufacturer, read their literature and press kits, perhaps snoop around their facility, spend hours searching the Internet, or review very boring government reports. *Eating Between the Lines* does all of that for you.

Sorting through and interpreting all the neon-loud messages, soft-spoken shelf talkers, ivory-tower-sounding brochures, and official-looking labels not only sabotages your family and play time; it can also have an impact on health. For instance, not long ago trans fats and hydrogenated oils were unheard of among consumers. Now scientific research and media reports offer plentiful warnings about the health danger of these sticky, heart-hardening fats. However, since there are some loopholes, reading the label may not be enough to understand the nuances. What about the low-carb and net-carb labels that are on everything from nutrition bars in the health-food aisle to mushrooms in the produce section? Once again, it will take the Food and Drug Administration (FDA) a few years to catch up with the marketers and offer guidelines about appropriate carbohydrate labeling.

Instead of a glossary of terms, this book is organized the way you shop, aisle-by-aisle. You can read the book like a power grocery shopping trip, from front to back, or skip around to particular chapters that match your shopping needs for the week. For instance, the first few chapters cover produce, meats, eggs, seafood, and dairy—the perimeter of the grocery store—where people shop most often. The remaining chapters represent the products of the internal aisles, such as the baked goods, canned foods, snacks, and beverages. This book is designed to help you make confident buying decisions while standing in any aisle at the grocery store.

The type of food one buys has become as prestigious as how you dress or to which school you send your child. Bad manners abound in the grocery store. I've tried to write this book as a guide, not as a judgment. Just before starting the book, I wrote an article for *The Denver Post* about how my family and I lived on food pantry donations for a week. I "shopped" at the local food bank for a week's worth of food, and my teenage son and I kept a diary of the experience. The rule was no eating out, no dinner or lunch invitations, and for my son, he could eat only the federally sponsored hot lunch at school.

By end of the week, I was sick, my growing teenage son was angry from being hungry all the time, and my husband, who is naturally thin, had lost weight he couldn't afford to lose. When we were down to only enough food for my husband and son, I went to the soup kitchen. The irony was I had just completed organizing a three-ton church food drive to distribute food to many of my lunch companions. They were kind and very open about sharing their plight.

The experience spotlighted how the best food is affordable to only the wealthy. It also made me realize that those who can afford such luxuries often judge the food choices of those who go hungry. The poor in my community are not the hopeless and homeless—they often work two jobs, shop at the same grocery store I do, and send their children to the same schools as my kids. They are also retired seniors living on fixed incomes.

The other marginalized group brought to light while I was writing this book was military families, who also rely on very limited incomes under very stressful situations. While writing I often thought of them and tried not to impart an unrealistic philosophy, such as "only buy organic," or "only buy from local farmers' markets," or "boycott certain grocers, like Wal-Mart." These are strongly held prejudices that can only be afforded by a slim margin of well-to-do individuals. My hope is that the book appeals to readers of all incomes, not just the lucky few who can afford to shop at the finest grocery stores.

If you are looking for a book that preaches to the choir about the value of sustainable food or tries to convince you that our farming system needs to return to the agro-centric days of a Jeffersonian lifestyle with a cow, a few chickens, and a garden in every backyard, or even that all our food should be purchased from sources of the like, this book is not for you.

While all of these ideas sound great in theory, once you get past the romance of rolling pastures and knee-high corn by the Fourth of July, much of the work to support such a lifestyle is shouldered by two-parent families, with large extended families who share the work. Today men and women working outside the home have to fit in carpools to soccer practice or dance class, private tutoring so their children can get into college, orthodontist appointments for picture-perfect teeth, perhaps a few moments of peace for a pedicure or to watch the news, and 17.2 minutes in the grocery store to track down something healthy for dinner and another 45 minutes to get it on the table—all between 3:00 and 7:00 P.M.

Personally, I have no desire to put up a season's worth of fruits and vegetables in canning jars, bake bread every Monday, preorder hindquarters of beef, pork, and lamb in the spring and fall and stash them away for the winter months in the freezer, and then resort to dried beans and onions in the dead of winter when nothing fresh is available from local farms. My great-grandmother, a farmer's wife, lived that way in Michigan fifty years ago, with the help of her husband, my dad, and his three strapping brothers—no thank you.

I like the convenience and selection of grocery stores. I like that I can find organic fruits and vegetables and naturally raised meats from reliable sources year round. Many of the so-called sell-out brands (Earthbound Farm, Coleman Natural Meats, Celestial Seasonings, WhiteWave, and Horizon Organic Dairy), which afford me this luxury, are being attacked for being no better than factory farms or that they are not organic or local enough (for me, four out of five of these are local Colorado companies, so "local" is relative to where one lives).

I can attest from writing about these companies since the mid-1990s that they didn't spring up overnight or skirt around food laws to gain their success. The founders spent decades building their brands, some forsaking their marriages, mortgages, and sanity, all for the cause—better-quality organic and truly natural foods. I don't begrudge them their success. In addition, these companies support hundreds of small family farmers who are grateful for once in their lives to have reliable incomes and a sense of financial security.

That said, when my budget allows, I indulge in purchasing a few pricier items at specialty and health-food stores. Better yet, from June to October there is nothing better than my town's local farmers' market. It's an important sector of our economy that deserves support (I serve on nonprofit boards to support school garden programs and sustainable farmers in Colorado). You may wonder what my cupboard looks like and whether I buy conventionally grown foods—absolutely. I do, however, think the conventional farming system needs updating—which, as you will read, is happening.

Eating Between the Lines is not meant to pit one food ideology against another—it is meant to educate. Which is why there are very few brands named in this book. Since there are tens of thousands of different products, too many to name, the overall goal of the book is to teach you how to discern important facts from any type of label, no matter the brand. Most of all, the book will help you recognize the ways of food marketers and to watch policy-making decisions with a critical eye. Often our government's attempts to mediate between the demands of a powerful food industry and the needs of the consumer leave the latter lost in the fray. Yolanda, where are you?

Eating Between the Lines

CHAPTER 1

Greener Acres Without Changing Your Address or Your Politics

Betting the Farm on Organics

"I am a farmer's daughter," I told myself again and again as I knelt on the ground, pushing away the soil to see if the green tint had faded from the pate of new spring potatoes. My sons, then five and two years old, stood by with a sturdy bucket and garden hose to give our bounty a good wash. We tugged at the wilting green tops, expecting to uproot clusters of walnut-sized starchy gems—instead, naked stems. We were stunned to be outsmarted by a sight-impaired mole, with a keen sense of smell. It, too, had patiently waited for the precise moment of agricultural perfection, and it had stripped our potatoes clean from the tops.

With looks of fortitude on their tiny brows, mud on their knees, and shovels perched on their sunburned shoulders, the boys took in their first farming lesson and headed to the back pasture to capture the thief. Our potato experiment came as a directive from my father, a Michigan farmer. "Buy organic potatoes," he said after hearing about a neighboring potato farmer whose kidney had shriveled to an unrecognizable mass. The suspected cause was decades of exposure to potent chemicals applied to his potato crops.

This was perhaps the first fatherly advice I can recall. While nearly all dads dish out dating advice to daughters, most of his paternal advice and our conversations edged around farming and food. After years of estrangement from divorce and what I call unpredictable family weather patterns, our tie was at times as deeply rooted as dandelions or as fragile and bitter as spring radish shoots.

But from season to season, no matter the family climate, his home-spun stories about his Midwest hundred-acre woods kept me fastened to a lifestyle that few ever experience in this urbanized society—the family farm. From an early age, my father learned that self-sufficiency was no farther than the backwoods. Orion was his lantern and the oak and maple his companions. As an adult, all he needed to fill the pantry for a year was a fishing pole, a garden, a hog in the pen, a dairy cow in the barn, chickens in the yard, grain in the fields, and a deer hanging in the shed.

He laughed at our potato-thieving mole and his tone let on that I finally understood, at least partially, the complexity and unpredictability of farming. Clever moles are just one of many problems potato farmers are up against. Beetles, blight, and fungus that can wipe out entire crops are common enemies, which is why this particular sector of agriculture has been so reliant on insecticides and fungicides—hence his advice to buy organic potatoes.

This was in the late 1980s, and I couldn't have told you what an organic potato really was or where to find them at the time, even though my address was in California's Central Valley, the nation's fruit, nut, and salad bowl. I had moved there from Manhattan and my prior zip codes included Washington, D.C., Hawaii, and London—all a far cry from my new rural residence. Perhaps my need to grow potatoes (along with peaches, plums, tomatoes, and cucumbers) was due to my desire to play catch-up. Conceivably, by playing in the dirt with my two boys I could make up on lost father-daughter years. Like reading through a family album of long-forgotten relatives in one afternoon, my hope was to learn about my familiar farming ancestry in one growing season; instead it's taken me more than twenty years.

In time, the navy ordered my husband to more suburban settings in Canada, Italy, and Colorado, but I didn't forget my father's advice. Still, organic vegetables were hard to find and the added expense wasn't something I could easily afford. For many years I was what the industry calls a cherry picker. If organic produce was on sale and within easy reach I bought it; otherwise there were no organic potatoes in my shopping cart.

It wasn't until years later, during my first job in journalism, that

I realized my father's down-to-earth advice did indeed have merit. I was thirty-five years old and working as an unlikely intern for a media and publishing company that served the health-food industry. The industry is known for utopian ideals and very liberal views. As I was a navy wife, my politics leaned toward the center and my wardrobe didn't include a single pair of Birkenstocks.

What's more, my relatives who made their living tilling the Midwestern soil were nothing like this breed of farmers. It seemed that all the organic supporters I interviewed staked their entire being on organic farming. For them it was a passion, almost a religion. Even my sister-in-law, who had lived in Seattle for decades, packed up and started a Community Supported Agricultural (CSA) farm in Mount Vernon, Washington. She farms as many as forty different items, including fruits, vegetables, eggs, and flowers, for her customers who collect their weekly share of food directly from Riversong Farm.

Why Buy Organic Produce?

Even with my loose ties to farming and my work in food journalism, which at the time was smack dab in the middle of the organic food revolution, I still needed pragmatic, methodical, Midwestern-style answers that transcended emotions. During some particularly tight financial months, the higher price for organic food was just too costly.

Most likely you've read, as I had, that organic fruits and vegetables are not subjected to pesticides. But why then were there newspaper headlines saying that organic foods had pesticide residues from chemicals like DDT? I'd been taught in journalism school, "If your mother says she loves you, check it out." I needed facts to justify a thinner wallet. Doubts, along with these questions, lingered in my mind each time I stood in the produce section:

- Was organic food really grounded in strong science or was it tethered by thin threads that could easily break when the next food fad came along?
- Are organically grown fruits and vegetables really better for my family?

- Did I fear being judged by coworkers, many of whom were single and didn't have a family to feed?

It takes a conventional farm three years to transition to organic; that's at least how long my conversion took. What changed my mind was a report by the Environmental Working Group (EWG), which was backed by the very independent Consumers Union (publisher of *Consumer Reports*). The list, called the dirty dozen, analyzed pesticide residue levels from the U.S. Department of Agriculture (USDA) government records. The no-nonsense list narrowed down the most common foods with the highest pesticide residues. Guess what? Potatoes were on the list. (I know, I should have listened to my dad.)

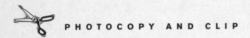 **PHOTOCOPY AND CLIP**

Fruit and Vegetable Pesticide Residues			
Most Residues		**Least Residues**	
FRUITS	**VEGETABLES**	**FRUITS**	**VEGETABLES**
Apples	Celery	Kiwi	Asparagus
Cherries	Potatoes	Mango	Avocado
Grapes, imported	Spinach	Bananas	Onions
Nectarines	Bell Peppers	Papaya	Broccoli
Pears	Lettuce (winter)*	Pineapple	Cauliflower
Peaches			Peas (sweet)
Raspberries			Corn (sweet)
Strawberries			

Sources: Environmental Working Group; USDA Pesticide Data Program 2003; Environmental Protection Agency

*Note: Winter lettuce isn't yet on the EWG list; however, preliminary EPA (Environmental Protection Agency) data show that perchlorate (rocket fuel) may be contaminating lettuce grown in southern Arizona and California, where 90% of the nation's lettuce is grown in the winter.

Finally, I had a manageable organic directory to work from. Instead of feeling guilty about not filling my cart with every organically available food and panicking that I was spending my kids' college funds, I now could use a workable list—one that fit my budget and relieved my doubts.

It's important to know that the residue levels on the dirty dozen are *after* these foods were washed and peeled for normal consumption. That said, I think (and hope) you can tell I'm not an alarmist. In general, the foods listed in the first two columns are higher in pesticide residues than others. However, to be fair and perfectly clear, the lists are not meant to imply the foods exceed EPA tolerable levels for male adults—it's the younger consumers who need more safeguards.

Very few foods ever exceed the EPA limits for adult males for three reasons. First, the agency must account for all pathways to exposure, such as diet, drinking water, and home use of insecticides, which means a piece of fruit is just one piece of the puzzle. It is the EPA's job to determine the health risk of each approved pesticide and set restrictions called tolerances, which is the maximum amount a particular pesticide can be in or on a food. The tolerance is not about pesticide residues; it is an estimate for one's exposure to a particular pesticide or its breakdown product.

Second, the EPA similarly looks at cumulative exposure to groups of pesticides that may cause cancer and considers all the ways we might be exposed, such as inhalation or through the skin. Third, the agency adds a 100-fold safety buffer when it applies the standards for pesticide residues.

Every year the USDA tests for pesticide residues on more than 13,000 samples, purchased at grocery stores, of fruits, vegetables, grains, milk, and drinking water (USDA Pesticide Data Program). In 2004, 76% of fresh fruit and vegetables showed detectable residues, 40% of these contained more than one pesticide, and only .2% exceeded the EPA's tolerable levels.

The EWG examines this same data and narrows it down to forty-six commonly eaten fruits and vegetables. The EWG dirty-dozen list is based on what is called pesticide load, which quantifies how many pesticides were found on a single fruit or vegetable and within the entire commodity. For instance, 92% of the apple samples contained pesticides; of those, 27% contained two pesticides, 24% contained three pesticides, and 12% contained four different pesticides. For potatoes, 79% contained pesticide residues, 52% contained one residue, and 21% contained two types of residues (this is a big improvement since my potato-farming experiment in the early 1980s).

The EWG list is significant, especially for pregnant women, infants, and children, because it raises awareness flags for foods that are commonly eaten by children and by moms-to-be during pregnancy. Ask parents of growing children and they will attest that kids eat a lot, and it's often the same foods again and again. In the 1990s reports began to emerge showing that the tolerable levels for pesticide residues may have been too lenient for kids. What was easily legal and tolerable for an adult male may pose an unnecessary risk to a child or unborn baby.

The issue was twofold: Pesticide tolerance levels had not been adequately analyzed for infants and children. Nor had science delved deeply enough into how low levels of exposure to certain chemicals could affect development. The presumption was that infants' and children's rapid rates of development and constant changes in metabolism could make them more vulnerable than adults to toxins, especially at certain times of development.

The National Research Council (NRC) called these potentially damaging opportunities "windows of vulnerability when exposure to a toxicant can permanently alter the structure or function of an organ system." The NRC goes on to say in their report "Pesticides in the Diets of Infants and Children" that "children may be more sensitive or less sensitive than adults, depending on the pesticide to which they are exposed," adding that there is no way to predict the infants' and/or children's sensitivity to these chemical compounds from data derived entirely from adults.

To right this anomaly, the Food Quality Protection Act (FQPA) became law in 1996. The law requires the EPA to identify safe pesticide levels for adults, children, and infants, as well as make regulatory decisions about new and widely used chemicals. The law required the

EPA to add a tenfold safety buffer to the already-established 100-fold safety factor when setting pesticide standards.

The first stages of the act required phasing out organophosphate (OG) pesticides, known to cause neurological problems in children if exposure is too high. Half of all pesticides used in foods eaten often by children are organophosphates. The effects from acute exposure to OG pesticides such as paralysis, seizures, and tremors are well-known. However, there were, and still are, no large human studies showing just how low-dose exposure to these chemicals interferes with children's central nervous system development. Rather than employ a wait-and-see approach, the FQPA called for reform.

The most common sources of OG pesticides are fruits, vegetables, and grains. Since the FQPA evaluation began in 1993 the amount of OG applications on all foods declined by 44%. The latest comprehensive reports show about 19% of all fruits, vegetables, and grains have detectable levels of OG pesticides, which is down 10% from the highest levels in 1996.

It's a good start; however, OG pesticides are still commonly applied to nearly half of the foods most frequently eaten by kids—including apples,* apple juice, bananas, carrots, green beans, oranges, orange juice, peaches,* pears,* potatoes,* winter squash, and tomatoes (* = on the dirty-dozen list). For the last federally released progress report of the FQPA, Consumers Union gave the agency a C— because of an organophosphate called azinphos-methyl (AZM). Among USDA apple samples from 2002, 37% tested positive for AZM. Apple juice and applesauce were considerably lower in residues (.1% and .6%, respectively, which suggests that processing may reduce exposure).

During the summer of 2006, the EPA submitted a proposal in the Federal Registry to begin phasing out use of AZM following a lawsuit filed by the United Farm Workers. Contradictory guidelines regarding the potent chemical put the EPA in a quandary when in 1999 the agency said that the chemical posed no risk to consumers or farmworkers. However, by 2001 research confirmed that farmworkers should not reenter orchards for as long as 102 days after AZM application, even though EPA standards allotted for a mere two weeks. Farmers who cultivate almonds, Brussels sprouts, pistachios, and walnuts will begin the phaseout in 2007. By 2010, apples, crabapples, blueberries, cherries, parsley, and pears will require less toxic alternatives.

The good news is that you can make a dramatic change in your child's exposure to pesticides now in a very short period of time. When children eat organic, as compared to conventional, foods the risk from pesticide exposure drops to well below what the EPA considers a negligible hazard to health. And by making the switch, you cause the levels and number of chemicals in the bloodstream to drop very quickly—within as little as seven days. The latest research shows that after one week of switching to organic foods, children's blood levels of common farming chemicals drop to negligible levels.

Overall, the FQPA has remarkable potential to substantially reduce exposure to pesticides, especially since diet accounts for up to 80% of exposure (the remaining is from water and home-use chemicals). Some states have taken the issue very seriously and have dramatically reduced pesticide and insecticide use through programs called Integrated Pest Management (see more later). For instance, in 1978 more than 201,000kg of pesticides were applied to potatoes grown in New York. By 1998 that level had declined by 52%, capping out at a little more than 52,000kg.

Busting the Myths About Organic Foods

If organic food were a Hollywood movie star, any publicity would be good publicity. But for organic food, there is a lot of noise from detractors drowning out some commonsense information. For many years I've watched the organic industry fend off verbal blows that say organic food isn't healthier. I've heard television reports state that organic food is more susceptible to dangerous microbes. And I've also read that it's just another fad that will soon pass. With each assault, dazed and bruised supporters stayed on task, steadily moving forward until they reached an economic momentum that the conventional grocery stores and food manufacturers couldn't ignore any longer.

For the first time, amid the Birkenstock crowd at health-food trade shows were suits with briefcases and clipboards. I'm certain these supermarket execs must have drawn straws to see who would attend;

this was, after all, foreign territory. At conventional food trade shows the most exciting spot was the beer tent, but here the stimulants and relaxants were herb based. When hunger struck, tofu hot dogs were plentiful, as well as whole-wheat pizza with dairy-free cheese. When trade show fatigue set in, massage chairs were at every corner, as well as aura readings for a quick karma check.

The new age wonders proved to be rich ground for conventional grocers. Grocery store profit margins are dismally small, only 1–3%, because of one overriding philosophy—grow lots of food and sell it at the cheapest price. This viewpoint, born out of America's post–WW II need to reduce malnutrition, was being challenged by a post-Vietnam generation that proudly boasted 20% sales growth for a food sector that was written off as a fad that only eco-minded hippies would support.

While the organic industry forged ahead, detractors stood in the back lobbing insults to weaken support for organic agriculture. The first assault targeted the conception that organic food wasn't any healthier, even though that was the common consumer belief. In the early years, the organic industry had no desire to prove such a claim; there were too many other mountains to climb, like USDA organic certification.

 Once USDA organic certification was approved in 2002 and this symbol began appearing on foods, researchers did indeed take the time to find that organic foods were higher in vitamins, minerals, and proteins (averages were higher in the following categories: calcium 63%, chromium 78%, iron 73%, magnesium 118%, potassium 125%, zinc 60%). The difference is due to a phenomenon called dilution, whereby nutrients in conventional produce have declined anywhere from 5 to 35% in the last fifty years because of pesticides, fast-growth fertilizers, and poor soil conditions. Since organic agriculture is as much a soil science as a food science, this news wasn't really that surprising to organic farmers.

Another attack cried fraud when a Consumers Union report tested conventional and organic produce for pesticide residues. The report showed that as much as one-quarter of organic produce showed some signs of pesticide residues. Never mind that many of the pesticides detected were long since banned, like DDT, which is still present in the soil and will most likely remain so for a very long time.

In addition, pesticides on conventional produce don't always stay where they are applied. These chemicals drift in the slightest of breezes and easily run off into the same groundwater used to irrigate organic crops. Know that while organic fruits and vegetables are not sprayed with synthetic and unapproved pesticides or herbicides, this doesn't mean they are completely free of any contaminants—they do, however, contain a fraction of what is seen on conventionally grown foods.

Also know that organic farming methods allow the use of common kitchen substances like mint oils and cloves to avert pests. In strong concentrations, even the most docile-sounding ingredients work effectively as pesticides. Organic agriculture also allows more potent substances, also considered pesticides, like *Bacillus thuringiensis* bacteria (Bt, the same bacteria, is inserted in genetically modified corn) and pyrethrum, a plant-based insecticide derived from the powdered, dried flower heads of the pyrethrum daisy. Even though these substances are allowed in organic food production, you wouldn't want to eat them, as they are naturally toxic. Nor would you want to dump these substances in the water or feed them to your pet, because they harm some wildlife. A perfect example is the controversy about the potential for genetically modified corn (Bt corn) to kill monarch butterfly larvae—nicknamed the Bambi of the farming world by *The New York Times*. While this might have been sensational news to nature lovers, this fact was not a big surprise to entomologists, who have always known that corn pollen exposed to Bt, organic or otherwise, will kill monarch butterfly larvae under just the right conditions.

Pesticides are designed to kill or at least repel pests, whether the substances come from your kitchen cabinet or a jar with a skull-and-crossbones danger warning. It's a matter of degree and scale. Critics of organic agriculture will use examples like Bt and pyrethrum to discredit organic agriculture. Know that pesticides are classified in four categories: highly toxic (class I), moderately toxic (class II), slightly toxic (class III), and relatively nontoxic (class IV). None of the thirteen pesticides allowed in organic farming exceed class III levels, and they are made from ingredients like bacteria and fungus, found in soil, flower petals, clay, and oils from plants. Conversely, conventional agriculture cannot make the same claim for the multitude of chemicals approved as insecticides and herbicides.

During the heaviest antiorganic stone throwing, few knew that most of the attacks were from an organization called the Center for Global Food Issues, a division of the Hudson Institute. It was founded by Dennis Avery, a supporter of biotech, who believes that genetically modified farming can help solve world hunger. Philanthropic efforts aside, the biotech industry has much to lose from the growing popularity of organic agriculture, since genetically engineered farming is prohibited for organically certified crops. Conversely, organic farming has much to lose from genetically engineered farming, because when a significant amount of modified genes drift into organic crops it can downgrade them to a conventional class, thus wiping out any chance of profit.

The Hudson Institute has the right to say and publish what it wants; just know where the motives lie. Also, know that each group threatens the existence of the other, which is why the attacks are so vigorous. You may remember the public apology from ABC News 20/20 coanchor John Stossel regarding a misinterpretation of data about bacteria and organic agriculture. Stossel and his staff were caught in a battle of words and wit going on for years between the Hudson Institute and the organic industry. It involved a myth that organic produce was higher in *E. coli* bacteria because of a lack of regulations regarding manure fertilizer.

Eventually, Stossel and others discovered that the *E. coli* reports were unfounded, hence the televised apology. To be sure, organic farming has a mandatory grace period for manure application and harvest—conventional farming does not. Since the Stossel debacle, reports show that manure on *conventional* crops may contribute to antibiotic resistance—something vegetarians thought they were protected from. It turns out that conventional manure may be tainted with the very antibiotics used in animal farming, which is exposing unwitting consumers to antibiotic residues that could reduce their ability to fight off infections.

This brings up the last point of organic certification—regulation and inspections. I know of no other industry that has asked so fervently to be regulated. For a farmer to be deemed a USDA organic-certified farm, the land must go through a three-year transition away from prohibited pesticides. During this time the farmer must adopt federally approved farming methods that include a variety of approved nonsynthetic fertilizers, antimicrobials, and biological-derived pest controls. Then the farm and the product are verified by an approved USDA third-party certifier. Only then can the food bear the green and white symbol.

This system is not without fault. In July 2006, *The Dallas Morning News* reported that the criteria for organic certification may not be enforced as strictly as has been promised by USDA. The article reviewed the 268 complaints submitted to USDA; 50 of these were for products that were not organic—although they claimed to be (the companies were ordered to stop). Also among the complaints were problems with overseas companies claiming to be organically certified, though perhaps they are not. These grievances are harder to enforce. For instance, the Beijing Consumers Association reported that among 268 organic food samples taken from city grocery shelves, 25 were counterfeit. Even U.K. consumers were shocked to see that pork and chicken labeled as organic and sold at shops on London's high streets were not actually organic.

Any certification system is only as good as its enforcement and oversight. Two events prior and post the Dallas newspaper report show positive movement in this direction. In the same summer as the Dallas newspaper story, the National Organic Program called for comments to tighten the certification parameters for imported organic foods. Just a week following the *Dallas Morning News* report, USDA revoked the accreditation for a third-party organic certification company, the American Food Safety Institute, in Chippewa Falls, Wisconsin, citing seven violations.

Food fraud is nothing new. Prior to the USDA organic certification rules, violations were common and inconsistencies in compliance from state to state even more so. In the mid 1990s, prior to the national standards, only seventeen states had mandatory organic certification requirements. Violations included selling conventional beans and grains as organic, dozens and dozens of farmers sold foods as organic when they were not, and one olive oil supplier went so far as to harvest olives from a golf course and label them as organic. In fact, a lack of consistency is one of the primary reasons a national organic standard was needed in this country. Above all, remember that the organic rules are new and the demand for such products is growing at a much faster rate than anyone predicted. The convergence of these two factors means that unethical opportunists will squeeze out whatever profits they can before they are caught. To add to the ruckus, as you will read in this book, there are the internal arguments within the organic industry about just how strict the organic certification rules should be.

If you doubt the severity of the rules, remember that when the first set of organic rules was released by the USDA, the organic industry and hundreds of thousands of supporters said the regulations weren't strict enough and asked for a reappraisal. Farming practices, like allowing sewage sludge to be used as fertilizer and using genetically engineered seeds, as well as allowing irradiation to kill harmful pathogens, were a few measures that quietly slipped into the original draft documents.

Since President Lincoln founded the USDA in 1862, no other issue than these three—sewage sludge, genetic engineering, and irradiation—has generated such passion and public comment. Luckily, Lincoln didn't have e-mail. Hundreds of thousands of organic supporters sent in e-mail and faxes criticizing the draft rules. Since the final rules were released in October 2002 there have been other attempts to loosen policies to satisfy less stringent agricultural desires, such as allowing for unapproved synthetics and nonorganic feed for livestock. As you will see throughout this book, each attempt to weaken the rules has been met with its fair share of comments, political activism, and consumer boycotts. So no matter what you may hear from critics, there is little reason to doubt the integrity of organic certification, because its own disciples won't tolerate ambiguities that allow for weakened standards.

Buy Locally; Thank a Farmer

At risk of family disownment, I will tell you that I still don't buy all my produce from certified organic sources. Buying local is just as important. Unless you live in Florida or California, it's not always possible, especially in climates like mine, with short growing seasons that are bookended between damaging spring frosts and heavy late-summer snows. However, staying true to local farmers, when possible, can precipitate big changes in the economic and environmental health of your community.

The grocery store has replaced any opportunity for urban and suburban dwellers to know much about the people who grow our food. Farmers' markets are our only opportunity to thank a farmer. Since the 1980s we've been told that the family farm is dying. Our first notion is that big farming is taking over, much like the mega–grocery stores that eat up any chance of survival for mom-and-pop corner grocers. In truth, the family farm is evolving much the way the rest of the country is, from single incomes to dual careers. Here is a snapshot of the family farm in the new century:

- Most farms in this country—as many as 98%—are classified as family farms.
- Small family farms gross $250,000 or less a year and account for about 91% of all family farms (about 6% are considered disadvantaged). They own about 70% of all available farmland, and as many as 82% of farms are enrolled in the federally funded Conservation Reserve and Wetlands Reserve Programs, which provide technical assistant for conservation farming practices and wetlands restoration.
- Large family farms account for 7% of all farms and gross $250,000 or more. Corporate farms represent 2–3% of farms overall.

Although small family farms are larger in number and own most of the land, they contribute only about 28% of total crop output. Large family farms produce about 58% of total crop output. Non–family farms account for 14% production.

As the numbers show, farm production is shifting from small

farms to large farms. The transition is occurring for two reasons: the number of retiring farmers outweighs the number entering the field, and profit margins continue to decline. To make up for smaller profits, as many as 40% of all small family farmers consider farming a second income. My dad, for instance, worked for the Michigan State Police and farmed on the side. Today he is supposed to be retired, but he hires himself out as a farmhand (he's as strong as any eighteen-year-old, more knowledgeable, and very reliable).

One way farmers are gaining notoriety and income is by selling directly and marketing through farmers' markets or grocers. Specialization is the key to survival. Entrepreneurial-minded farmers are selling high-end products like grass-fed and organic pork and beef, specialty fruits and vegetables, and organic dairy products for higher margins than conventional crops because they can set the prices rather than rely on commodity prices.

Although the portrayal of the small family farm is shifting, the total value add from farms of all sizes to a state's well-being is as significant as that of a large factory or corporation. For instance, in Iowa farmers' markets alone contribute as much as $33 million in sales and additional economic activity to the state. Combine this with the monetary contributions farmers make to the tax base, added with the revenue from commodity farm sales and related small businesses, and most communities would collapse without the farms' presence—not to mention we would be very hungry.

If you need another excuse to buy local beyond supporting your local community, think about its impact on the earth. I would like to leave a smaller oily footprint on the pavement when I hand life's baton to my grandchildren—buying food from local sources can make a big blow to pollutants.

Let's stay in the same state, Iowa, to prove the point. A University of Iowa study looked at seven foods and how far they traveled to get to Chicago, the distribution hub in the Midwest. The researchers limited the fruits and vegetables to domestic and Mexican produce— squash and pumpkins had the lowest mileages at 781 and 233 miles, respectively; sweet corn 813 miles; apples 1,551 miles; asparagus 1,671 miles; broccoli 2,095 miles; and finally grapes at 2,143 miles.

These seven foods collectively traveled 9,287 miles, the same flight distance from New York City to Sydney, Australia.

The second phase of the study measured emission reductions and fuel consumption for twenty-eight Iowan-grown foods versus foods shipped in from afar. Fuel emission reductions were as high as 8 million pounds, and fuel savings reached as high as 346,000 gallons. The truly amazing find was that the study's food sample size represented only 1% of the total consumption for Iowans—though the impact on emissions was equal to removing sixty-five cars from the road. So while you may think the only way to help solve the current fuel situation is to walk or to buy a hybrid car, buying locally grown food whenever possible can make a huge difference in our dependence on oil imports.

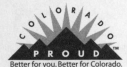 Most states have USDA-supported local buying programs for fruits, vegetables, and other grocery products. In my state, it's Colorado Proud, as noted by this symbol. Each state has its own logo and marketing program. One worrisome trend in farmers' markets is to allow vendors to truck in products from outside the state and even the country. This type of competitive pressure can easily put local small farmers out of business. If you see such practices in your own farmers' markets, voice your opinion until someone listens.

My only warning about the newly founded interest in buying local is that there is criticism that organic food that is trucked in or flown in isn't organic because of the food miles. As I mentioned earlier, food miles matter, but only Californians and Floridians can live year round on only locally produced food. In other climates, such as mine, winter tables would be limited to pinto beans, popcorn, potatoes, onions, apples, and pumpkins—no thank you. For those of you who are fortunate to have local foods all year long—*bravo!*—but let me buy my California organic lettuce and Florida oranges in January from the supermarket.

Letting Go of Supermodel Food

You may have to get over the eye-candy factor when buying local food from farmers. For supermarkets it takes a great deal of commitment from the management to buy local fruits and vegetables. Their first priority to the consumer is a regular supply of fruits and vegetables that meet a certain eye appeal.

America's obsession with visually perfect food often prejudices our opinion about what good food looks and tastes like. Here's an example of how wasteful it has become. Years ago, while attending a grocery store food conference in Baltimore, I stole away for a morning field trip to a local farm. My traveling companions were African farmers here to learn about the American grocery market. The farm was a model of sustainability—no chemical pesticides or herbicides, and mounds of vines, leaves, tomatoes, and squash were piled high between the rows for organic compost. The farmer had a comfortable contract with local health-food stores to supply vegetables.

The farmer kindly allowed us to harvest a few tomatoes to take back to our hotel rooms. While I picked through the vines, the African visitors reached into the compost pile for perfectly fine samples. The farmer embarrassingly explained that these weren't fit for the store because they weren't the right size. Too polite to question the farmer, our guests waited until we filed back to the bus to ask why these glorious specimens were thrown away. We responded timidly with no good answer.

Buying local often means turning a blind eye to fruits and vegetables that are perhaps not uniform size or lack the shiny wax coating that makes them glimmer under the hip halogen lights in the produce section. Even if a vegetable isn't the Gisele Bündchen of the tomato world, good looks don't always mean the best flavor or the most nutrition. Get over this; the difference in taste is dramatic. You won't need much convincing after biting into a Colorado peach, Washington apple, or New Jersey tomato that has traveled only a few miles to your kitchen.

Produce Labeling

ECO-FRIENDLY LABELS

USDA Certified Organic   Farming is the manipulation of the environment to suit man's need for foods. It's been happening since Stone Age man discovered how to grow grain for food. The level of exploitation has waned and waxed since the end of WW II when new chemicals emerged from advances in war technology.

Today organic agriculture seeks to manipulate the environment in the least damaging manner by prohibiting most conventional pesticides and fertilizers made with synthetic ingredients or sewage sludge, as well as prohibiting bioengineered species and irradiation. Before a product is labeled USDA-certified organic, a third-party government-approved certifier inspects the farm for compliance. Be wary of produce stands and vendors at farmers' markets that claim their fruits and vegetables are pesticide-free; there is no such valid claim—either a farm is certified organic or it's not.

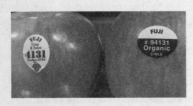

You'll have to read the fine print to find organic certification on produce. The traditional green organic seal doesn't fit easily on lumpy green peppers or velvety mushrooms, so suppliers place the Price Look Up (PLU) code on the packaging, on a sticker, or directly on the produce with a laser tattoo. Conventional produce has four digits, usually starting with a 3 or 4; organic has five digits, beginning with a 9; and genetically modified (GM) fruits and vegetables have five digits and begin with an 8.

If you are wary of GM fruits and vegetables, rest assured that you won't find many examples in the produce section, yet. Patents exist for potatoes, summer squash and zucchini, radicchio, tomatoes, and papaya. However, with the exception of papaya, each time the USDA has tried to move crops from the experimental phase to production, it's been met with such opposition that few crops have succeeded commercially. A GM tomato, the FlavrSavr brand, was sold in supermarkets from 1995 to 1997, but it was a financial bust. A few farmers have attempted to grow GM summer squash, but they, too, have had trouble convincing the public to buy it.

Genetically modified papaya is the only fresh GM food that has any long-term history in the fields and the store. About half of Hawaii's papaya crop is genetically modified, a move that rid the plants of a damaging virus called papaya ringspot. Supporters say the gene modification saved the papaya industry from demise. Non-GM papaya growers are concerned the gene will drift to their plants, limiting the number of available products for organic customers, especially for overseas clients. Unless you live on the West Coast or in Hawaii, it's not likely that you've seen GM papaya, because most papayas are imported from Brazil, Mexico, and the Caribbean, according to a study by Cornell.

 Certified Naturally Grown   The Certified Naturally Grown (CNG) label is for farms that grow produce using at minimum the USDA organic standards but have sales of less than $5,000 per year. The CNG label follows the same labeling guidelines as the USDA organic seal, but it's more applicable to smaller farms that grow more than one crop. Look for the label at a grocery that buys local produce, as well as on fruits and vegetables sold at farmers' markets, CSA farms, local restaurants, co-ops, and small grocers. CNG randomly tests 10% of its members' products for pesticide residue to ensure the integrity of the program.

 Biodynamic Farming   This nongovernmental certified farming program declares the entire farm as sustainable and biodynamic. The rules are more stringent than those of organic food production for pest and weed management, crop rotation, composting, as well as water and energy conservation. Harvesting follows a moon calendar, which means you may see biodynamic farmers on their tractors in the moonlight. The principles of biodynamic farming were established by Rudolph Steiner; followers adopt an overall lifestyle that supports their environmentally conscious growing methods and interest in following the natural growing seasons. This means you won't find fresh peaches in December or just-picked apples in July that are certified biodynamic.

Integrated Pest Management   I don't mean to pick on potato farmers; they have had a tough time with the low-carb craze. It's just that potatoes are particularly prone to pests and diseases, which is why pesticide and fungicide use is prevalent. A farming system called Integrated Pest Management (IPM) is turning the conventional potato industry around in a very positive direction. IPM uses old-fashioned farming methods, like those my grandfather taught my dad, such as soil preparation, well-timed planting to reduce infestation, frequent scouting and pest trapping, introduction of beneficial insects, as well as a definition of a clear threshold of infestation before a pesticide can be applied. IPM doesn't mean absolutely no pesticides or fungicides, just less. A Consumers Union study, using 1998 and 1999 data, showed what you might expect: the order of highest to lowest levels of pesticide residues were conventional, IPM, and organic. Today as many as 37% of potato growers have IPM programs, or better, in place.

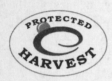

One of the most noted IPM programs involves a collaborative effort by the Wisconsin Potato and Vegetable Growers Association, the World Wildlife Fund, and the University of Wisconsin. Through a shared interest in cleaning up Wisconsin's potato industry, farmer participants reduced toxicity indexes by as much as 50%, especially for pesticides considered very toxic. Protected Harvest also certifies California IPM-grown strawberries, as well as California wine grapes. Protected Harvest also has grants to expand to dairy, almonds, tomatoes, and stone fruit in the Central Valley in California, which will begin in 2007.

There are varying degrees of IPM; some are more ecologically minded, while others have been nicknamed "Improved Pesticide Marketing," a phrase coined by Rex Dufour regarding the number of disparate IPM definitions. Ideally, IPM should mean, "ask questions first and spray later, but only as a last resort." But since IPM is not a government or third-party certified farming method, the decision about when to apply pesticides can be too hasty or suitably reserved, depending on the commitment by the farmer. The most stringent IPM method endorsed by Dufour is called bio-intensive IPM (BioIPM), which recognizes the same methods as more conventional IPM programs; however, the threshold for pesticide application is higher with bio-intensive methods.

The IPM system is a good one, one that should be visible in more grocery stores. It accepts the reality that not all farmers can or are willing to go completely organic. The biggest fault is the lack of a single list of prohibited substances allowed on crops and uniform oversight— there have been dozens and dozens of different definitions of IPM since its inception during the Nixon administration in the 1970s. When the concept was first introduced the goal was to convert as much as 75% of American farms to IPM; however, today the scope is somewhere between 4 and 30%. It wasn't until the last five years that the USDA even began setting goals and desired outcomes to define IPM as a marketable farming practice.

The most well-supported IPM consumer labeling program, sponsored by Wegmans grocers in New York, is a perfect case of demand outstripping supplies. In 1997, the company began an IPM certification program in cooperation with Cornell Cooperative Extension and the New York State Department of Agriculture & Markets for its private-label fresh, canned, and frozen fruits and vegetables. Unfortunately, the program is on now on hold as a victim of its own success. A company spokesperson says the IPM program isn't defunct; it's temporarily on hold until more producers sign on. Another victim of lack of support was the Massachusetts "Partners with Nature" IPM marketing program, which lost funding from the Massachusetts Department of Food and Agriculture in 2000. The program had operated for six years, with as many as fifty-one growers.

Dufour says the biggest barrier to acceptance of IPM programs is pressure from chemical companies, especially for farmers who lack the type of historical knowledge that is often passed down from generation to generation or at least a close relationship with local farm bureaus. It's not too surprising that farmers who rely on crop management advisers apply as much as two-thirds fewer pesticides as farmers who turn solely to chemical companies for advice. He says that often chemical company salesmen will serve as pest control managers—but since their paycheck depends on selling chemicals there is some conflict of interest in the relationship, a problem my father has witnessed all too often.

Dufour manages a USDA-sponsored free phone hotline and online resource for farmers who grow organically or simply want to convert to more sustainable farming methods, but the chemical salespeople are persistent and seem to always be available, he says. "Somewhere along the way, the concept of IPM was hijacked . . . ," says Dufour, "and drifted away from ecological pest management."

The leading detractor for change is the true potential for, or fear of, crop loss. It wasn't until 2000 that Congress passed a bill to improve crop insurance coverage for farmers who choose IPM farming methods. The incentives for farmers to change to IPM practices are multifaceted; however, without adequate support and cold, hard cash from supporters other than chemical companies, there may be little incentive for the farmer to take such a risk.

WASH BEHIND YOUR CORN EARS: FOOD SAFETY LABELS

Produce isn't the first food category that comes to mind for food-borne illnesses, but from 1990 to 2003 it was the leading cause, with 25,823 reported cases, outnumbering poultry by more than 13,000 and beef by almost 15,000, according to the numbers from the Center for Science in the Public Interest.

The cases include *E. coli* in bagged greens, salmonella from sliced tomatoes and cantaloupes, hepatitis in green onions, and parasites from raspberries. The sudden rise in illness has upped the awareness of microbes in convenience foods like bagged and presliced produce, and food scientists are working to correct it. For instance, you may notice that bagged lettuce resembles a plastic blowfish. This is from modified atmosphere packaging whereby ozone is pumped into the bags to prevent bacterial buildup. (See the Addendum in the back for additional information on spinach and *E. coli*.)

Fresh foods pose a greater risk for illness because we are eating more of them, which is a habit we shouldn't change. The other reason for the increase in illness is that more fruits and vegetables are imported from across the globe, where the standards for clean water irrigation and health and safety procedures may be less stringent.

One solution is awareness and traceability through mandatory country-of-origin labeling for produce, which has been met with strong opposition from food associations and has yet to be approved. There are behind-the-scenes improvements including good agricultural and manufacturing practices for all sectors of the supply chain and a traceable audit system, which emerged from new laws designed to protect food from bioterrorism—not food-borne illness.

At present, the only visible consumer warning is a result of government-supported "Fight Bac" education campaign with this clever character. The best protection is to wash your hands with soap and water before and after handling fruits and vegetables and follow these guidelines:

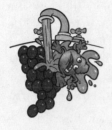

1. Don't buy bruised fruits or vegetables, and cut out any visible blemishes.

2. Rinse produce under running water, including those with skin and rinds that are not eaten. Rub or scrub firm-skinned produce with a clean vegetable brush, under running tap water.

3. Do not use detergent; water is fine. Vegetable washes are designed to remove wax, but they aren't antibacterial. Statistics show that washing fruits and vegetables under running water will remove some, but not all, pesticides from the skin.

4. If you are a high-health-risk individual, such as a person with an autoimmune disease or one who is undergoing chemotherapy for cancer or chronically ill, wash all fruits and vegetables—even if the label says prewashed. The FDA says that bagged, ready-to-eat produce need not be washed; however, one of the recent illness outbreaks involved bagged prewashed lettuce, so be aware.

5. Dry produce with a clean towel.

6. Keep produce separate from raw meat, poultry, and seafood in your shopping cart and at home. If produce comes in contact with raw meat or fish, throw it out.

7. Refrigerate all cut and peeled or cooked fruits and vegetables within two hours or throw it away.

8. Throw away any bruised and damaged portions of fruits or vegetables that will not be cooked. If in doubt, throw it out.

Bottom Line

In recent years the EPA has begun the monumental task of removing some of the most toxic pesticides that have built up in our farming system and soil since the 1930s. The agency is paying better attention to the vulnerability of children to pesticide residues, but there is still work to be done.

While detection is not an indicator of health risk, the pesticide residue levels still raise concern. Environmental toxicologists say 80% of all pesticide exposure over a lifetime is from our diets (water and residential exposure accounts for the remaining 20%). Therefore, changing one's diet can be the single easiest way to reduce exposure. Now that organic foods are so readily available in grocery stores, you won't have to resort to growing your own as I once did.

The excuse of cheap food at any cost isn't supported any longer by consumers. It would be a good day if the only two choices consumers saw in the produce department were IPM and organic. Unfortunately, IPM has not been marketed as well as organic, namely because it isn't a single entity with monitored guidelines. For a successful program, one that consumers can trust, IPM needs the same government commitment and third-party certification for growing methods and finished products as the organic industry. The Protected Harvest IPM program is a good starting point.

There are other changes that need to take place before you will see any absolute and radical changes in the system, namely, interest from consumers and farmers. The chief reason the organic industry is growing at more than 20% a year is plain ol' profits. Yes, organic agriculture decreases exposure of pesticides, and yes, it is better for the environment. But now that organic agriculture and food production has moved past being a burgeoning cottage industry into mass markets, profit is the driving force. In other words, if we don't buy organic and IPM foods in quantities large enough to support the bottom line, neither will survive.

It will take a different kind of cajoling to convince conventional farmers to at least switch to IPM. The organic industry was founded by pure emotion and passion, while conventional farmers are grounded in more conservative rural values and are less willing to risk it all for a new world order. In the organic industry when activist groups called for boycotts and verbal assaults to attack the farming industry as a whole, organic farmers and like-minded consumers responded. But these tactics only make independent, salt-of-the-earth conventional farmers dig their clay-caked boot heels farther in the dirt. The most successful IPM programs are those that use cooperative partnerships, instead of bashing, as is witnessed by the Wisconsin Potato and Vegetable Growers Association and Protected Harvest collaboration. This pesticide reduction program based itself on not only the knowledge of conservationists but also the wisdom of conventional farmers and field-wise experts from farm bureaus.

Last, farmers need some guarantees and protection while making the conversion, such as better-funded research and crop insurance. Few consumers realize that farmers work on such slim margins that they have little room to maneuver and that financial ruin is at times as close as the next bend in the road. Let's take one last look at potatoes as an example. In 2000, the average consumer price for a ten-pound bag of potatoes was $3.80—the farmer saw $.66 of that; the remaining $3.14 went to packers and storage businesses, marketers and retailers. Of the $.66 the farmer saw, more than half, $.37, paid for the seeds, land, water, equipment, fertilizer, pesticides, and labor. This leaves the farmer with a $.29 profit—if yields are down and pests are up there are few options to change the status quo. Farmers say the money to come up with new techniques has to come from somewhere other than their well-worn pockets—like wealthy food processors and USDA-sponsored research grants, not chemical companies. It's time for the detractors to stop slinging the manure—organic is here to stay—IPM needs better support at the government, retail, and consumer level.

CHAPTER 2

Slaughterhouse Semantics: Beef, Pork, and Lamb

What Should "Natural" Beef Really Mean?

A passing comment at the Coleman family dinner table in 1979 compelled Colorado rancher Mel Coleman, Sr., to redefine the beef industry. Daughter-in-law Nancy Coleman innocently suggested to Mel that he market the type of beef that was set aside for the family freezer—beef raised without hormones or antibiotics and range fed. "Natural," she said.

The word "natural" would lead this cowboy down a path he never expected. The trailhead began at the Sangre de Cristo Mountains in Colorado and cut straight to the bureaucracy of the USDA, the politics of the meatpacking industry, and, after much hardship, ended in grocery stores nationwide when the words "natural beef" became as commonplace as the Golden Arches. He once told his biographer that his was "just another ranch and cowboy story." Don't believe it.

This Colorado native grew up doing what his father did, raising cattle in the San Luis Valley, near the town of Saguache (pronounced SA-watch). The town slogan at one time was, "We've got plenty of nothing." To valley cattle ranchers, nothingness means a high, wide berth of arid grasslands, the valley's most valuable natural resource. The Ute Indians named the region Saguache for the "water at the blue earth." Mountain streams that percolate at the Continental Divide filter down to the valley's blue-green earth floor. It's just enough water to nourish the grand cottonwood trees that cling to the stream's edges and mark homesteaders' claims like the one Mel's great-grandparents staked in the 1800s.

Mel knew how to run a cow-calf operation, the first stage of beef production, but he didn't know much about raising cattle from the ranch to table, as his daughter-in-law recommended. In the traditional supply chain, cattle change hands numerous times before reaching the final feedlots. Mel was proposing one long vertical progression, unfettered by growth hormones, antibiotics, and multiple owners. Cattle would graze 20% longer to reach their weight rather than be involved in a race toward rapid weight gain in crowded feedlots. It was novel, but to Mel it was how his father raised cattle before the advent of growth-promoting hormones and antibiotics.

In the early 1980s, Mel sold natural beef from the back of a pickup truck to anyone willing to listen to a cowboy with a fresh supply of ranch stories and a cooler of beef. Mel knew that marketing natural beef would be contentious because the portrayal compared the powerful conventional beef industry to this new breed. "But I didn't see that as a problem," Mel said in his biography, *Riding the Higher Range: The Story of Colorado's Coleman Ranch and Coleman Natural Beef* by Stephen M. Voynick (Glen Melvin Coleman, 1998). "I had no intention of selling natural beef at the expense of the regular beef industry. I planned to offer natural beef only to consumers as an alternative product. The consumer would be the judge."

It was a hard sell at first. Mel started marketing juicy slabs of natural beef at health-food stores in Boulder and Colorado Springs but was met with skepticism and downright revulsion. At the time, health-food stores catered to mainly vegetarians. Mel measured his success at health-food trade shows by "how many brochures ended up in the trash."

All Americans, not just health nuts, were leery of beef, a fear brought on by reports of illegal implants of diethylstilbestrol (DES) in as many as 427,000 cattle. DES, a human drug used to prevent miscarriages and premature deliveries, was banned in the early 1970s when physicians discovered it caused reproductive cancers. The drug was also a valuable growth promoter for cattle until it was banned in 1979. Even so, feedlots in twenty states continued to use it the following year. The FDA investigation and media coverage of the corrupt and dangerous practice gave Coleman Natural the boost it needed to keep going.

But it was a decision by the USDA in 1984 that revealed the beef industry and government's real opinion of the maverick company. Eighteen months earlier Coleman won USDA approval for a "natural beef" label; it read as follows: *Feed used is always hormone and stimulant free. No artificial or synthetic ingredients. Only minimally processed. USDA does not permit preservatives in this product.*"

There were other products on the market that said "natural," but none could prove it. Coleman's label was backed up by a paperwork trail detailing every step. This solid start in traceability would serve the company well in later years when other crises like mad cow disease battered the beef industry. Officials at the USDA gave Mel confidence to think that the agency would continue to use this definition of "natural" from then on.

Not so. In a surprising move, the USDA downgraded the definition of "natural" to mean any meat that was "minimally processed and contained no artificial ingredients." Mel recounted in his biography, "The USDA addressed only the meat, but we addressed the animal *and* the meat. I argued that you can't give animals hormones and antibiotics for their entire lives, and then say the meat is natural. But the USDA wouldn't listen. They bowed to pressure from the regular beef industry, which wanted to get rid of me and the other natural beef producers."

When Mel Coleman passed away in February 2002, the company had overcome much debt and doubt to become the leading natural beef company. Mel's story lives on in his son Mel, Jr., a tall, sturdy man with his father's mischievous eyes and smile, as well as his commitment to natural beef. Mel, Jr.'s cowboy boots, starched shirt, and firm handshake say a lot about his roots. Just like his father, he would like people to think he's just another Colorado cowboy, but now, as the chairman of Coleman Natural Foods, Mel, Jr. has taken up his father's charge to get a true definition of natural beef, not the watered-down USDA version. Mel, Jr. calls it staying "true to the trail" his father blazed.

Mel, Jr. is pushing the USDA to agree to his father's definition of "natural," one that prohibits the use of antibiotics and hormones. Even for a company that pioneered a strict definition of "natural" and "hormone- and antibiotic-free" beef, Coleman admits getting that message to consumers is still a tough trail to forge.

Should I Worry about Mad Cow or Let It Go?

In March 2006, the third case of mad cow was reported in this country. On the very same day, in the very same breath that the USDA confirmed the test results, the agency announced that the bovine spongiform encephalopathy (BSE) surveillance program was winding down from 7,000 cows a week to a mere few hundred. This was perhaps the most poorly timed announcement in recent food history. In addition, Agricultural Secretary Mike Johanns said to the press, "Testing is not a food safety measure. Rather, it's a way to find out the prevalence of the disease."

Tact and good timing apparently aren't strong suits for the agency. Although technically BSE testing is a measure of whether the disease has infiltrated our farming system—not our hamburgers—the declaration was a poor way to gain consumer trust. Has the USDA gone mad or is the risk for mad cow truly on its last legs?

The decision comes down to numbers, one three-digit number in particular—173. This is the sum of the unaccounted cattle that were shipped to this country from the U.K. before the 1989 import ban (all E.U. cows were banned in 1997). According to data collected for a Harvard Risk Assessment, 334 cattle were imported from the U.K. during 1980–1989, before our country banned the use of ruminant-to-ruminant animal feed in 1997. All but 173, of the original 334, were accounted for.

The Harvard study concluded that at the highest point of vulnerability no more than 24 of these cattle might be infected with BSE. When researchers added other values to the equation, such as mortality, feed bans, restricting beef by-products in animal and human food, the risk for BSE spread dwindled further, down to as few as 4 to 7 cattle as of 2006.

If one looks at this country's history, undoubtedly there isn't even a hint that a BSE epidemic is circulating in the U.S. food system, as the tragedy seen in Britain. Looking back, political foot dragging played a role in the E.U. crisis, but so did variables that couldn't have been foreseen. In his book *Brain Trust*, Colm A. Kelleher, Ph.D., a cell and molecular biologist, unravels the many unimaginable events that led to the crisis.

Aside from the now well-known cause of animal feed made from ruminant animals, Kelleher describes an unpredictable catalyst—a 1974 industrial accident at a British solvent manufacturer that killed 29 people and injured 100 more. The disastrous outcome forced the imposition of safety controls on all businesses using inflammable solvents, one of which was the animal-rendering industry for animal feed.

Rather than upgrade to the more expensive safety standards, the rendering companies chose to forgo using the solvents. While this was a perfectly legal option, no one suspected that the solvents aided in the extraction of infectious BSE proteins from the final product, thus helping reduce the spread of the disease. The BSE spread climbed exponentially higher when U.K. rendering plants upgraded to more efficient processes that not only increased production but also caused BSE to spread.

These small changes, coupled with ten years of incubation, passed before the first visible BSE case in a British cow was reported in 1985. By 1993, more than 100,000 cattle were infected. Meanwhile, it would take even more time to convince U.K. ministry officials that there was an undeniable link between BSE and the newly discovered human illness vCJD (variant Creutzfeldt-Jakob disease). The first human deaths were reported in 1995, but admission of the new disease wasn't until 1996. It took twenty-two years after BSE unsuspectingly entered the food supply for government and industry officials to put all the pieces together, and by then the U.K. beef industry lay in ruin, leaving too many grieving families in its wake.

The insidious nature of this disease always leaves room for uncertainty. Even the Harvard researchers, who ran the numbers on every possible scenario in the farming system, couldn't predict whether humans would develop vCJD. The researchers dared only to foretell the predictability in cattle. Human risk adds another layer of complexity that is next to impossible to predict, which is why some have called for mandatory BSE testing of all cattle.

Thus far, any attempts by individual states or companies to adopt their own testing programs have been shut down by the USDA under the guise that such entities lack authority to conduct their own programs. The USDA and the National Cattlemen's Beef Association fear that false positives could lead to widespread consumer panic, as well as higher costs that could lead to more volatility in the marketplace.

Many of the beef companies petitioning to independently test their products want to do so because they export their beef to Japan, which temporarily banned U.S. beef imports because of sloppy mistakes in quality control. Often, Japan is held as the model program since they test all cattle for BSE. Although testing is extensive, it isn't often noted that Japan didn't implement feed bans until 2000, when its first case of BSE was reported. To make up for lost time and to gain consumer confidence, a 100% testing plan was developed. From this vantage point it looks like the icon of testing perfection. However, with the passage of time, as Japan's risk has declined, even they have begun to scale down their testing program.

The USDA has stood firm that this country's feed ban, which was implemented in 1997, and the import restrictions are the strongest barriers to transmission. The assurance may have held up until Canada announced its fifth overall BSE case in the spring of 2006, from a cow born *after* the feed ban. It was the second of this type (a sixth case, from a fifteen-year-old cow, was reported a few months thereafter). The United States buys most of Canada's cattle for beef production. The very same week as the sixth reported case, Canadian agricultural officials announced that it would prohibit the use of cattle tissue suspected of causing BSE from all animal feed, pet food, and fertilizer, effective July 2007. Canadian beef shipments to the United States were suspended in 2003 and resumed in the summer of 2006 for cattle younger than thirty months. USDA officials said they made that decision with the knowledge that more Canadian cases would be reported.

Food safety watchdog groups fear that this is another example of why the feed industry needs even tighter controls, especially for feed rendering. Given that the U.K. disaster was precipitated by an unforeseen catalyst—a change in cleaning fluids—Consumers Union was quick to comment that this country's feed ban is only as good as the enforcement. The Center for Science in the Public Interest wants the FDA to require feed machinery and even entire mills to be designated for specific species to prevent cross-contamination.

To add to this unease, in June 2006, the USDA announced that the two most recent BSE cases in Alabama and Texas were an abnormal form of the disease. Suspected causes included contaminated feed and a spontaneous BSE manifestation. Another theory from veterinary disease specialists is that the cattle contracted this atypical BSE from a similar neurological disease in sheep called transmissible spongiform encephalopathy (TSE), more commonly known as scrapie (scrapie does not transmit to humans).

Since BSE testing began in June 2004 only two cases were verified among the 350,000 randomly tested cows. The USDA Office of Inspector General (OIG) notes that the lack of detection may be because the inspection system isn't specific enough. The OIG believes that the USDA may be looking in the proverbial wrong haystack. Instead of random tests, the OIG suggests focusing on old cows, born before the feed bans. In addition, the OIG recommends increasing inspection rates to hot spot regions, like the Pacific Northwest, where many Canadian-born cattle now live (the Northwest had the lowest sampling percentages of the six regions).

Clearly, as the OIG suggests, there are still loopholes in the system. Then again, the overall risk for BSE spread is dwindling. The Harvard study that predicted the spread of BSE from the original 173 unaccounted cattle estimated that without any further provocation it takes about twenty years for BSE to completely diminish from the cattle population. Just when this twenty-year period ends depends on the starting line. If the starting point is 1989, when the U.K. import ban went into place, it's about another two years. If the starting point is 1997, when the feed ban was implemented, it will take another decade to reach the twenty-year finish line.

In March 2006, the United Nations' Food and Agriculture Organization (FAO) reported that BSE had declined to 474 cases worldwide (down from 878 in 2004 and 1,646 in 2003). The number of human deaths from vCJD was 5 in 2005, 9 in 2004, 18 in 2003.

If the numbers aren't enough to ease your mind, there are a few measures you can take at the grocery store to reduce the risk even further.

First, know the beef's source. BSE incubates for a long time, usually manifesting in six to eight years. The three cases reported in this country were from older cows born before protective feed measures were in place in 1997, which means know the source of your ground beef. Hamburger made from old dairy cows poses the most risk. There is even less risk if one buys beef from cattle that have eaten only grass and grain, with no animal by-products (as they are born to do). Labels like "beyond natural," "grass-fed," and "organic" will point to this practice.

Second, understand that BSE resides primarily in the spinal cord, brain, small intestines, and tonsils, not muscle tissue. So avoid sweetbreads, bone marrow, neck bones, beef cheeks, and cuts sold on the bone. Also, purchase ground beef rather than hamburger. Some grocers grind their own ground beef. Also, ground beef is made from specific cuts (i.e., ground chuck, ground round, or ground sirloin). Hamburger is made from multiple cows, from trimmings and less popular cuts of meat. Remember, cooking does not kill BSE.

Third, buy from suppliers that have a tracking system in place. In early spring of 2006, the USDA introduced an animal-tracking system for bison, poultry, dairy cows, cattle, and swine (a system already existed for sheep and goats). The announcement came just after the latest case of BSE from a cow in Alabama. Although the animal never entered the food supply, USDA inspectors were not able to track down the ten-year-old cow's original herd to see if other animals or offspring may have also been infected. (The USDA said it's unlikely that more than one animal per herd, or more than one offspring, would be infected.)

By the time the tracking system is fully implemented in 2009, the National Animal Identification System will assign each participating animal an electronic ear tag, which will allow it to be traced back within forty-eight hours. The limitation is that the program is voluntary. It's too early to predict how many suppliers will come on board (as of April 2006, 235,000 ranches and farms were registered, out of

800,000). Some small beef suppliers have had systems in place for many years; it's not a bad idea to seek out these suppliers. Currently, Canada and Australia have mandatory ID systems in place.

Last, think about buying bison for ground meat; it makes great burgers. Bison are not susceptible to BSE, laws prohibit animal by-products in feed, as well as antibiotic and hormone use, and it's very lean. The most medication a bison will ever receive is a vaccination to prevent a wasting disease also seen in elk and deer.

Safe Handling

"Put me out of business, please."
—WILLIAM MARLER, SEATTLE TRIAL ATTORNEY

The preceding quote is heartfelt and honest. Although Marler has a successful career, he'd just as soon find something else to do. This trial lawyer represents some of the worst cases in this country—kids getting sick from food. In Marler's world, there are no winners. His clients are grieving parents who have lost children to food-borne illnesses or are nursing desperately sick children. He is particularly bereft about the state of the ground-beef business. Marler has been calling for changes to put him out of business. Since he made that plea in 2002, some improvements have come about. Let's see how it's going.

1. **IMPROVEMENT:** In January 2002, a rapid detection system was introduced that identifies *E. coli* in five minutes. Inspectors can identify the problem immediately—long before it's entered the food supply. In addition, a new rinse-and-chill system using sterile water, mild acids, and salts (lactic, acetic, sodium chlorite—the same salt used for contact lens cleaning) is being tested to reduce *E. coli* and salmonella in ground beef.

2. **IMPROVEMENT AND SETBACK:** Tests from the Food Safety and Inspection Service (FSIS) affirm that *E. coli* contamination rates are

down by 43% since 2003. However, in 2005 nearly 1 million pounds of hamburger and ground beef were recalled for *possible* *E. coli* contamination. Statistically it's a small percentage when compared to the more than 7.5 billion pounds of hamburger and ground beef consumed each year, until one considers that this is the equivalent of 4 million quarter-pound hamburgers.

3. **IMPROVEMENT AND SETBACK:** The current system of meat recalls is voluntary. No company has ever refused to recall a contaminated product, but companies can delay recall announcements. Any holdup means the tainted food has more time to reach the consumer's plate. Public comments are under way to allow an easy-to-access list of retail locations for recalled meat, so consumers can pin down where and when they may have purchased a recalled product.

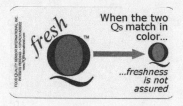

4. **IMPROVEMENT**: This label is a good use of wartime technology. Originally developed as a sensor for homeland security, these highly sensitive labels detect when food spoils and send out a message to the shopper to leave this package on the shelf. The labels, called FreshQ, change from a fresh tangerine color to gray when the meat is spoiled. Look for it on beef, pork, and chicken.

5. **IMPROVEMENT AND SETBACK:** The FDA allows for carbon monoxide gas in beef packaging to help the meat maintain a bright red color, called Modified Atmospheric Packaging (MAP). While there is no evidence that the process is harmful, it can mislead consumers into thinking that a product is fresh when it may be well past its sell-by date. Consumers Union tested MAP-packaged ground beef and found that two of the ten packages were spoiled and one was almost spoiled, but the meat was still vividly red.

The American Meat Institute defends its use, saying it's no different from MAP processes used for bagged lettuce, peanuts, potato chips, and cookies. This statement isn't exactly accurate.

MAP technology for potato chips, peanuts, and cookies uses nitrogen; lettuce, carbon dioxide—and none of these products spoils as rapidly as meat.

Meat turns brown for two reasons—when a protein called myoglobin loses oxygen (MAP prevents this) or when the meat spoils (MAP doesn't prevent spoilage). Therefore, don't rely on meat color for a safety gauge; read the dates on the package. Wal-Mart, Kroger, Publix, Stop & Shop, A&P, Wegmans, and Whole Foods are among those to have banned meats that use carbon monoxide.

The City Council of Chicago considered passing an ordinance to ban the practice for beef sold in city stores; as of press time, the proposed ordinance was reduced to mandatory labeling. If you are wondering why MAP technology may be a setback as well as an improvement, according to a University of Georgia study MAP-treated beef may apparently be lower in *E. coli*. Untreated meat that was inoculated with the pathogen had twelve times as many *E. coli* cells. I caution you to still read the packaging dates. *The New York Times* food editor Marion Burros once left a package of MAP-treated beef on her kitchen counter for a week—it kept its youthful red hue for the entire seven days.

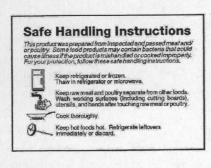

Safe Handling Instructions

This product was prepared from inspected and passed meat and/or poultry. Some food products may contain bacteria that could cause illness if the product is mishandled or cooked improperly. For your protection, follow these safe handling instructions.

Keep refrigerated or frozen. Thaw in refrigerator or microwave.

Keep raw meat and poultry separate from other foods. Wash working surfaces (including cutting boards), utensils, and hands after touching raw meat or poultry.

Cook thoroughly.

Keep hot foods hot. Refrigerate leftovers immediately or discard.

SAFE HANDLING INSTRUCTIONS

Bacteria such as *E. coli* are present on only the surface of muscle cuts, such as steaks and roasts. Grilling or searing kills any surface bacteria. Ground beef is another issue altogether. During production, contaminated particles hidden within the intestines can come into contact with beef in the grinding process. The bacteria churn through the ground meat tainting everything in their path. For this reason, if Marler has his way, the warning label would say something like *"This product may contain animal feces that could cause illness if the product is cooked below 160 degrees."*

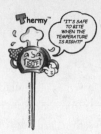

Since it is doubtful such a label will ever exist, the primary rule in ground-beef safety is to cook it to the recommended safe temperature of 160 degrees, particularly for children and the infirm and elderly. In addition, cook or freeze ground beef within two days of purchase to prevent the spread of harmful bacteria.

One solution that has been highly supported by the beef industry is irradiation. It is currently available for fresh or frozen ground beef, hamburger and patties. Please remember that irradiation *will* kill bacteria at the meatpacking plant. It's a long way from there to your table. Critics feel strongly that the label gives consumers a false sense of security because irradiation cannot prevent microbes from spreading during transport, at the store, or at home. Therefore, treat irradiated beef with the same care and safe handling as regular ground beef.

Beef Labeling

NATURAL AND ORGANIC BEEF LABELING

USDA Definition of "Natural"   "Meat that is minimally processed and free of additives such as preservatives, artificial flavors, or colors" is how the USDA defines "natural." It's a processing claim and has nothing to do with how the animal was raised. For consumers, the only type of meat that doesn't qualify for this definition is meat that is marinated or has an added solution to the finished product.

Beyond Natural   There are no well-defined government-sanctioned parameters for natural beef beyond the USDA's very broad description. For the lack of a better word, truly natural beef companies do not administer antibiotics, ever; do not use hormones, ever; and forbid synthetic pesticides, always. As equally important, these ranchers use conventional grains with no animal by-products in the feed. The primary difference between these brands and organic is that the feed is certified organic in the latter case. To reduce costs, "natural" beef companies use noncertified grass and grain and the range/pastureland isn't certified organic. Whole Foods, Wild Oats, and health-food stores require all meat sold in their stores to be raised at the very least with these types of standards.

How the producer goes about raising "natural beef" varies. Most natural beef companies have ownership of their cattle from birth to slaughter. There are exceptions. For instance, some companies contract with ranches that agree by affidavit to follow similar guidelines. To keep the ranchers accountable, the company tests the cattle for residues. If residues are detected, the animal is removed from the supply. Needless to say, this method is controversial within the natural beef industry because complete control along chain of custody cannot be guaranteed.

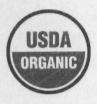

USDA Certified Organic   Beef that meets the USDA National Organic Program (NOP) standards must be fed 100% organic feed; no hormones are allowed, ever; no antibiotics, ever; and no synthetic pesticides, ever. If antibiotics are ever necessary, the cattle are removed from the herd and sold elsewhere. The animals may have been pasture fed for their entire lives or during the last 120 to 200 days have been moved to a finishing lot where the diet is organic silage and grain that contains no animal by-products.

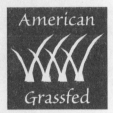

Grass-Fed   These cattle eat grass their entire lives, never entering a corn feedlot. There are reports of grass-fed beef with so-called "minimal feedlot exposure." There is no such thing—grass-fed means only grass-fed. The American Grassfed Association (AGA) is hoping for USDA-approved certification program to prevent such deceptions. To date, there is only one grass-fed livestock certification program, in Marin County, California.

In May 2006, the USDA proposed a grass-fed label—the proposed standards weren't strict enough for the AGA, so the language is being worked out. According to the AGA, "grass-fed" should mean the cattle are fed only pasture grass and silage (dried cut grass). The only give in the rule is 1% nongrass feed to allow for inadvertent feeding of nongrass (i.e., if the cattle decide to stick their head through the fence to partake of something other than grass), but nothing more. There are discussions about whether grass-fed certification should allow antibiotic and hormone use—there are opinions on both sides.

But until there is a federally approved label, the term "grass-fed" can mean just about anything. The best advice until a firm definition is approved is to buy from producers who are members of the AGA, a consortium of grass-fed beef companies (they represent beef, bison, dairy, goats, poultry, and lamb). If you prefer brands that are not treated with antibiotics or hormones, look for certified organic or beyond natural grass-fed beef brands.

The health advantage of grass-fed beef is higher levels of vitamin A and vitamin E and increased levels of omega-3 and conjugated linoleic acid (CLA), a healthy fatty acid depleted over time from the food supply as farming methods changed from grazing to increased time in feedlots.

Vegetarian-Fed   This label means the cattle are fed grass and grains. This is perhaps the most underutilized label in the meat counter, though it has the biggest implications. Vegetarian-fed cattle are almost free of risk for contracting BSE because their supplemental feed is not made from rendered animal by-products. As a stand-alone label, vegetarian-fed doesn't have anything to do with hormone or antibiotic use.

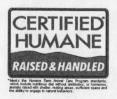

Certified Humane   This program is overseen by Humane Farm Animal Care, which is funded by organizations including the American Society for the Prevention of Cruelty to Animals (ASPCA), the Humane Society of the United States (HSUS), and humane societies throughout the United States. USDA verifies the inspection process to make certain that growth hormones are prohibited and the animals are raised on a diet free of animal by-products and antibiotics in feed. The animals must be raised in adequate space and in a manner that allows natural behaviors. Processors must comply with the American Meat Institute

Standards, a higher standard for slaughtering farm animals than the federal Humane Slaughter Act.

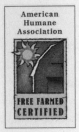

Free Farmed This label means the product is certified by the American Humane Association (AHA). You may be familiar with this group's work to prevent child abuse and its oversight of movie and television sets to make certain that animal actors are treated safely. The association's certification process for livestock monitors the conditions for food, water, shelter, and grazing space, as well as the manner in which the cattle are shipped in railcars and handled for slaughter. The AHA also monitors cosmetic companies that agree not to use animals for cosmetic product testing.

Biodynamic Farming Biodynamically farmed beef is sold seasonally, as the farming principles are based on nature's rhythmic seasons. This means if you want to buy biodynamic beef, you'll have to buy it at or near June to stock up and freeze it. The pedagogy of biodynamic farming is decades older than organic agriculture. It's based on the teachings of Rudolph Steiner, and "seeks to actively work with the health-giving forces of nature." If you are truly committed to local, chemical-free beef that has been raised and butchered using very strict principles, this is for you. It won't be easy to find because of the commitment by its farmer followers to following the seasons, so plan ahead.

BEEF GRADING, ORIGIN, AND FAT CONTENT

The inspection and grading of meat and poultry are two separate programs within the USDA. Safety inspections are mandatory; grading is not. Veterinarians from the FSIS oversee inspections of live animals. As mandated by the Federal Meat Inspection Act, the FSIS also inspects raw beef for microbes and chemical contamination. State inspection programs are at least equal to FSIS standards.

Beef grading is a voluntary paid service for meat producers. The grades are based on standards for quality—prime, choice, select, and standard.

Prime   The highest-quality grade. The tender cuts are rich with butterlike marbling, which stands up well to dry-heat cooking, such as roasting, broiling, and grilling. Prime is often reserved for restaurants and catering.

 Choice   This meat has less marbling than prime and is more readily available at the grocery store. Roasts and steaks from the loin and rib are very tender and also hold up well to dry-heat cooking. Less tender cuts include rump, round, and blade chuck and should not be overcooked.

 Select   Has less marbling than and is therefore leaner than choice or prime. Loin, rib, and sirloin can be grilled, broiled, or roasted. For the best flavor, do not overcook. Other cuts should be marinated or braised for tenderness and flavor.

Standard and Commercial   These grades are often sold ungraded or as store brand meat. Retired dairy or breeding cows are generally slaughtered between six and eight years of age. Their tougher meat is usually sold ungraded as ground beef or used in processed products.

Branded Beef   A brand is not a grade of quality; it's a marketing program. The brand might be a breed of cattle or a marketing campaign; examples are Certified Angus Beef, Steakhouse Choice Premium Angus, Cattleman's Collection, and Rancher's Reserve. The standards for quality and aging vary from brand to brand. I'd like to compare them for you, but it's proprietary information. Some of the branded beef is labeled as prime, choice, or select. The marketing goal is to entice the consumer with brand loyalty, not necessarily beef grades.

Country of Origin   U.S.A. Beef, Fresh American Beef must be from cattle born, raised, slaughtered, and processed in the United States, or in a specific state. When beef is labeled as "Processed in the USA," that means the cattle were slaughtered and processed in the United States, although the cattle may be imported from elsewhere.

Another anomaly in this labeling tactic applies to other meats, such as lamb. Lamb imported from another state or country may be labeled as, say, "Colorado Lamb," as long as it was finished, slaughtered, and processed in the state.

American Wagyu beef is from a Japanese-bred steer that is now raised in this country (similar to Japanese Kobe beef). The grading system is a Japanese numbering system that ranks marbling from 1 to 12. According to the Kentucky Beef Council, American-raised Wagyu scores between 5 and 8, as compared to USDA prime cuts, which are graded as a 4.

GROUND BEEF AND HAMBURGER FAT CONTENT

You might think that ground beef and hamburger are the same; think again. Hamburger has added fat, as much as 30%, to stretch out the weight; ground beef does not have added fat. Should you pay for all that fat? While it can add flavor, much of it cooks out. Broiling will reduce the fat content in 30% fat hamburger from 35g of fat (per three-ounce serving) to 18g. If you blot the cooked patty on a paper towel for thirty seconds, the fat content will drop down to about 11g. Personally, I'd rather pay more for the meat than the fat.

Most inexpensive ground beef is 30% fat and 70% lean. Single cuts of beef are also ground and sold as ground chuck, ground round, and ground sirloin. Each will vary in the amount of lean meat and fat by cut, but in general from highest to lowest fat content it's hamburger, ground beef, ground chuck, ground round, and ground sirloin.

It's important to note when reading a ground-beef label for fat calories that the official USDA serving size for ground beef is three cooked ounces (just less than four ounces raw), not a half-pound burger, as is often seen on restaurant menus.

In addition, if you see a label that says "70% fat-free hamburger," this does *not* mean it contains just 30% of its calories from fat. It means the product is 30% fat by weight, which can add up to a lot of fatty calories. Look for *extra-lean* meats because they contain less than 5g fat and less than 2g saturated fat per three-ounce serving. Extra-lean cuts, of all types of beef, include eye round roast and steak, sirloin tip side steak, top round roast and steak, bottom round, top sirloin, brisket (flat half), and 95% lean ground beef.

Pork

There is a little-known fact about the pork industry: hormones are not allowed for growth promotion—so any label that says "no hormones" is making an obsolete point. Pigs' highly sensitive systems are susceptible to many diseases, especially when pigs are housed in close quarters. To combat the resulting health problems widespread applications of antibiotics have been the easiest solution. This practice has been criticized by consumer groups because of its contribution to antibiotic resistance in humans and waste runoff that pollutes groundwater.

Researchers have been watching farmers in Denmark since the country banned the use of antibiotics in all animals to prevent disease. Unfortunately, the ban for pigs wasn't as successful as that in other industries, like bans on antibiotic use for broiler chickens or hens. The pigs got sick, which only increased the amount of drugs used to treat illness. The solution is apparently broader than just limiting drugs.

The National Pork Board, the industry's trade association, will try to overcome its reputation for being too freehanded with antibiotics when it releases a new program and respective logo (the graphic was not available at press time) for pork products raised under the PQA (Pork Quality Assurance) Plus program in June 2007. The program seeks to reduce the need for antibiotics with sound basic standards for herd health, such as housing that is warm and comfortable and reduces stress and better weaning practices that reduce susceptibility to disease.

Liz Wagstrom, D.V.M., assistant vice president of science and technology for the National Pork Board, describes pig farms as being like day-care centers for children: "For the first three months of preschool, it seems that children attract every little germ. It is the same for just weaned pigs, especially when the farming system offers little opportunity for them to build resistance." Wagstrom explains that in the past, farming procedures didn't take this into account and, rather than adopt a wait-and-see attitude, antibiotics were often applied too soon and too often.

The PQA Plus program is a voluntary program that will offer training and guidelines for judicious uses of antibiotics, as well as good nutrition and biosecurity measures to reduce disease outbreak. "It is diagnostics, rather than guesswork," she says. Before the label is released, as much as half of the pork industry is already participating in an education program called Take Care, Use Antibiotics Responsibly to reduce antibiotic use. The PQA Plus program expects an even higher involvement rate, but it's too soon to report on compliance. Wagstrom says the pork industry is taking responsibility for what it can control, rather than adopting an "it's not my problem" approach, as in the past.

In 2005, Compass Group, a major food supplier for hospitals, colleges, restaurants, and catering, announced that it will no longer purchase pork that is treated with growth-promoting antibiotics. The company's supplier, Smithfield Foods, promises to report its total usage of antibiotics and continue to reduce use over time, without raising prices. We can only hope that this trend will spill over to the grocery sector and other producers.

BEYOND NATURAL PORK

Producers that use no antibiotics and label their products as natural face the same challenges as the beef industry. The USDA definition of natural pork means the product is "minimally processed and cannot contain any artificial flavor, color, chemical preservatives, or any other synthetic ingredient"—however, it is often difficult to distinguish between the USDA definition of natural and a more stringent definition.

Beyond natural pork suppliers focus on methods that are similar to but not as extensive as organic livestock methods. They rely on alternatives to human-grade antibiotics, avoid growth-promoting drugs, and provide spacious pens for confinement and grain feed, as well as using safe waste management systems. Generally, as with other brands for natural beef, the animal feed is not always organic.

Omega-3 Enhanced Pork   Designer pork chops, rich in heart-healthy omega-3 fatty acids—who would have guessed? There are two ways animal scientists are testing this theory. One is by feeding pigs a diet rich in flaxseed; the other is a bit more sci-fi and not likely to show up in stores just yet. Scientists protracted a gene, called the fat-1 gene, from roundworms and reprogrammed it to convert omega-6 fatty acids (something we get too much of) to omega-3s. Since the science uses genetically modified animals, the FDA will have to get in on the approval process, which is a long way off. In the meantime, a Canadian company using the flaxseed model began marketing their products last year. To get the maximum benefits, one must eat the fat, because it holds most of the essential fatty acids—there is no word yet on what cardiologists think of the new product.

Organic Pork   Pigs that meet the USDA NOP standards must be fed 100% organic feed, no antibiotics, ever, and no synthetic pesticides, ever. If antibiotics are ever necessary, the hogs are removed and sold elsewhere.

To date, there are only a few organic pork producers that supply products nationwide. Most consumers equate antibiotic resistance with poultry products; however, utilizing a supplier that uses no antibiotics in pork can have a significant outcome in reducing incidence of antibiotic resistance and the harmful environmental impact of standard hog-farming practices.

Free Farmed and Certified Humane   Both of these certified programs are similar to the programs described earlier for beef. The pigs are raised with clean bedding and space to roam; growth-promoting drugs are not allowed. Many of these farms raise rare breed stocks, which result in pinker, rosier-colored meat than the traditional "other white meat." Both programs also monitor for humane slaughtering methods.

Biodynamic Farming   Although some of the lifestyle choices of biodynamic farmers have been mocked, biodynamic pig farming creates an environment that the conventional pork industry can only wish for—a disease-resilient pig farm. These pigs raised among other animals and grown to full weight at a slower pace thrive and are virtually free of disease. If problems do arise, biodynamic pig farmers use homeopathic therapies. As with beef, the pigs are butchered seasonally—pork season is the fall.

SAFE HANDLING

You may recall your grandmother telling you to cook pork until it was well done, often to a scorching and dried-out 180 degrees Fahrenheit. The precaution was to eliminate a disease-causing parasite, *Trichinella spiralis*, which caused the illness trichinosis. Improvements in feed practices since the 1950s have practically wiped out the risk of contracting the parasite. You have a better chance of getting the illness from eating wild bear, cougar, and wild boar (the only pork-related cases have been from home-grown meat), so unless you eat roadkill or live off the grid, there is little worry.

In all honesty, the meat only needed to reach 137 degrees to kill any parasites; however, the USDA is obligated to say that cooked pork should reach a temperature of 160 degrees to kill off other microbes like *E. coli*, salmonella, staphylococcus, and listeria. How one reaches this internal temperature, if at all, depends on your cooking style and your opinion. While rare pork is not very tasty, many professional chefs and home cooks serve pork medium (between 140 and 150 degrees), cooked to a rosy pink hue. Whichever temperature is your preference, take the meat out of the oven or pan when it is five degrees below the desired result, cover, and let it sit for about ten minutes to allow the temperature to continue rising.

PRODUCT DATING

Product dating is not required for pork. If you see a sell-by date, use or freeze the product within three to five days of purchase. If it's a use-by date, follow it.

Lamb

Lamb is produced from animals less than a year old, and baby lamb is marketed at six to ten weeks old. Spring lamb is processed from the first Monday in March through the first Monday in October. The term "spring lamb" was important decades ago when lamb production peaked in the spring and lamb purchased in other seasons was usually sold frozen. Today this term is almost obsolete because of year-round processing.

In most grocery meat cases you will find only two grades of lamb, prime and choice. Lower grades of lamb and mutton, from older sheep, are seldom sold in stores. Prime- and choice-grade lamb is sold as chops, roasts, shoulder cuts, and leg. It can be cooked with dry heat by broiling, roasting, or grilling. Less tender cuts, such as breast, riblets, neck, and shank, should be cooked slowly and braised in liquid.

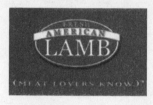

American Lamb   This label is a marker of origin for U.S.-raised lamb; the leading states for American lamb are Texas, Wyoming, Colorado, Utah, and South Dakota. As much as 73% of lamb is imported to this country, most from New Zealand and Australia. If you wish to support American-raised lamb, look for this symbol. American lamb generally weighs more at processing than imported lamb, so the cuts will be larger. This label is a marker of origin, not a certifying label regarding livestock-growing methods or organic practices.

Free Farmed and Certified Humane   These are the same programs as for pork and beef. The lambs are not subjected to growth hormones and growth antibiotics. In winter months the feed may be fortified with hay and grain. Processors with the Certified Humane label must comply with the American Meat Institute Standards, a higher standard for slaughtering farm animals than the federal Humane Slaughter Act.

Grass-Fed Lamb   As with other meats, certification for grass-fed lamb has been proposed. Grass is the natural diet for sheep, although many sheep ranchers supplement with feed grain because American consumers prefer meat that tastes less gamy. The advantage to only-grass-fed lamb is abundant omega-3 fatty acids and conjugated linoleic acid, both heart-healthy fats. Since there is no officially monitored definition yet, some grass-fed lambs are just that—only grass-fed—while others are supplemented with grain to accommodate the American palate. The American Grassfed Association is working to rein in this type of marketing.

Organic Lamb   The biggest obstacle to buying organic lamb in the United States is availability. USDA organic standards prohibit the use of certain antiparasitic drugs that fight off a common stomach worm; some importing countries do not. Organic sheep growers have a less potent arsenal of options, which are more expensive than conventional treatments. If you happen to find USDA-certified organic lamb it will not have been subjected to parasitic drugs, antibiotics, or growth hormones and will have been raised under humane conditions.

Bottom Line

Ever since cowboys saddled up the to bar to pay for a shave, a shower, and a thick steak, cattle drives and the old West have been blazoned into our American persona. Carhops and ponytailed teens on roller skates popularized the hamburger in the 1950s, and since then advertisers have asked, "Where's the Beef?" and told us, "It's What's for Dinner."

Most recently, the beef industry never had a better friend than the high-protein Atkins diet. After twenty years of declining beef sales, the protein-packed diets gave permission for repressed beef lovers to openly admit their admiration for a steak or a burger. In tandem, the beef industry developed cost-efficient feedlot raising methods to slim expenses and promoted beef as an affordable, healthy, and quick meal for time-starved families, thus pushing sales up by an average of 12% from 2000 to 2003, the equivalent of about $1 billion per year.

It's all working, because consumers barely flinched when prices rose sharply because suppliers were caught off guard with the heightened demand or even with reports of the first case of BSE in North America in December 2003. It's understandable that a flawless system isn't realistic for every cattleman or meat packer. Thanks to action by the USDA, the risk for BSE remains low in this country. Still, a carefully designed tracking system and a carefully monitored animal feed supply are mandatory for human and animal health. The belief that it can't happen here is naïve, whether it's *E. coli*, BSE, or some unforeseen food safety threat.

If demand for specialty beef is any indicator, the beef industry should be paying attention to consumer demand. In 2006, there were shortages for natural, organic, and grass-fed beef. Perhaps it's time for the USDA to listen to Mel Coleman, Jr., and others like him to come up with a true definition of natural beef. It would satisfy consumer interest for beef raised outside the traditional system, and practices like fewer hormones and no animal by-products in feed might rub off to the conventional beef industry. Like Mel Coleman, Sr., said, "Let the consumer be the judge."

FREE-RANGE BEEF AND BISON

"Is this bison free-range?" This is a common question that friends of mine hear at the Fort Trading Company, sellers of bison and Coleman Natural Beef. Let's get something straight—all bison are free-range. If you've ever seen these magnificent beasts you will understand why. In fact, other than the white man's shotgun, the barbed-wire fence was the bison's (then known as the buffalo) greatest enemy. Yes, bison roam free and eat grass; they may get a little grain. The only drug bison ever receive is a vaccination at birth to prevent a cruel wasting disease that also sickens wild deer and elk.

In addition, all cattle are free-range or pastured for most of their lives. It isn't until they reach a large enough size for a feedlot that they are brought in (about 1,100 pounds or more). See the "From Range to Plate, the American Beef Industry" on pages 50–51.

From Range to Plate, the American Beef Industry

You may question why certified organic and brands positioned as beyond USDA's definition of natural beef cost more, so here is a timeline for how the cattle industry is run. The first line is certified organic and beyond natural beef; the second line is conventional beef; the third line is grass-fed cattle (which can also be certified organic, beyond natural, or conventional). The primary differences are in the use of hormones, antibiotics, and nonvegetarian and corn feedlots to reach maximum weight in a shorter time period, hence the cheaper price. Beyond natural, organic, and some-grass-fed brands allow more time to reach the maximum weight and have a less potent arsenal of drugs to treat disease—which costs more.

ORGANIC, BEYOND NATURAL

"COW CALF"	7–9 MONTHS	"WEANER or STOCKER"	15–16 MONTHS "FEEDER"	16–24 MONTHS	30 MONTHS
I------I		------I------		------I------I------II	
75 pounds	500–600 pounds		800–900 pounds	1100–1300 pounds	Slaughter
Grass, hay, range		Range, pasture	Winter wheat, corn stubble, grass, grains	Grains, roughage, silage	

------NO ADDED HORMONES, ANTIBIOTICS------→

CONVENTIONAL BEEF

"COW CALF"	7–9 MONTHS	"WEANER or STOCKER"	15–16 MONTHS "FEEDER"	16–24 MONTHS	30 MONTHS
I------I		------I------		120–160 days	
				------I------I------II	
75 pounds	500–600 pounds		800–900 pounds	1100–1400 pounds	Slaughter
Grass, hay, range		Range	Corn/soy, protein/carb feed	Corn/soy feedlot	
		Hormones*(very limited)	Hormones*(common)	Hormones*(common)	
		Therapeutic Antibiotics†	Therapeutic Antibiotics†	Subtherapeutic Antibiotics* and Therapeutic Anitbiotics†	

GRASS FED‡ (CERTIFIED ORGANIC, BEYOND NATURAL BRAND, OR CONVENTIONAL)

"COW CALF"	7–9 MONTHS	"WEANER or STOCKER"	15–16 MONTHS "FEEDER"	16–24 MONTHS	30 MONTHS
I------I		------I------		------I------I------II	
75 pounds	500–600 pounds		800–900 pounds	900–1100 pounds	Slaughter
Grass, hay, range		Range/pasture	Range/pasture, grass		

* For growth (there is a forty-five-day grace period before slaughter for hormone and antibiotic withdrawal)
† For disease
‡ American Grassfed Association rules allow for a 1% nongrass feed, as long as it is inadvertent, for instance, where the animal forages on something other than grass such as wheat or corn stubble. Until there is an agreed-upon definition, grass-fed allows for all types of raising methods, including conventionally used hormones, whose members believe hormones shouldn't be allowed, as is true for bison.

CHAPTER 3

Hatching Profits: Chicken Labeling

Tastes Like Chicken, but Is It Hormone-Free?

I tried to ignore it, but I couldn't help it. There it sat—chicken, lots of it, all neatly stacked in the grocery cart in front of me. The red, yellow, and blue packaging caught my eye among the baby lettuce, heirloom apples, soy smoothies, and organic blue corn tortilla chips.

Confrontation is not my strong suit; still I blurted out, "Why do you buy that brand of chicken?" Twenty years ago, the man attached to the shopping cart might have taken it for a pickup line; instead, today he looked offended, and rightfully so.

I live near Boulder, Colorado, where what one eats defines a person as much as his or her house, clothes, or car. Boulderites are passionate about health, fitness, and environmentalism, including organic agriculture. Stand on any street corner and you'll likely hear a group of people, just finishing an afternoon run, discussing what to do for dinner—perhaps dining at a sustainable restaurant or grabbing something at Whole Foods or Wild Oats.

So, as one might imagine, this handsome, ponytailed Teva and Patagonia–clad twenty-something man looked at me as if I had accused him of the worst possible crime. When he realized I wasn't going away, he admitted, "My wife tells me to buy it. She says it's healthier because it doesn't have added hormones."

"None of them do," I said, "but that costs more than other brands." He bought the chicken anyway; naturally it was safer for him to listen to his wife than a nosy stranger in the checkout line. Sir, whoever and wherever you are, consider this a public apology for my behavior. After all, you were listening to your wife—a commendable, although ill-informed, decision.

I could name drop and tell you the brand, but it's irrelevant since all hormones were banned in poultry operations in the late 1950s. Not that they didn't try it. After trial and error, producers discovered that hormones create soft chicken meat and don't help much with growth during a chicken's short life span.

This little-known fact hasn't kept producers from trying to convince you that their chicken is superior because it has no added hormones. Marketers are smart enough not to put "hormone-free" on the packaging, since the USDA won't allow it unless there is a disclaimer about the prohibited use. The rider doesn't make for very compelling labeling copy, but since the Federal Trade Commission (FTC) isn't as stringent about its enforcement, the "No Hormones" claim makes for very profitable advertising.

Don't buy into it. The real sham is that niche companies charge as much as three dollars more per pound for essentially the very same product other, conventional producers offer. Don't be fooled; remember that no poultry operations, large or small, use hormones. Therefore, the labels "No Added Hormones" and "No Added Steroids" are simply reiterations of a policy that exists for all poultry producers—so don't pay more for hormone-free chicken.

Who Is Playing Chicken with Our Health?

What my labeling-shopping victim and his wife really want is chicken labeled as "Raised with No Antibiotics." These chickens have never, ever been given antibiotics. This shopper's quest will require a bit of detective work, because although it could be profitable, most conventional grocers don't carry this type of chicken. Instead, diligent shoppers have to look for it in health-food stores, co-ops, and specialty stores (Super Target recently added a no-antibiotics brand).

It's a common mistake to mentally string words like "antibiotics" and "hormones" together, as if they were one and the same. Smart poultry marketers count on this. After all, few of us took Poultry 101 in school. Marketers know that in the instant it takes you to make a buying decision, you will most likely not make the mental distinction between antibiotics and hormones.

In the poultry industry, antibiotics *are* used for growth promotion, as well as disease treatment and prevention. At issue is that the same drugs prescribed by your doctor are the very same drugs poultry farmers can use to fatten up their chickens and turkeys, as well as prevent and fight off diseases. The overabundant use of antibiotics on the farm and in human medicine creates a vicious cycle called antibiotic resistance.

The first point to remember is that antibiotic resistance has nothing to do with antibiotic residues. Since all poultry are required to undergo a withdrawal period after being given antibiotics, it's not the antibiotic drug residues passing from chicken to humans that pose a health risk. It's the antibiotic-resistant DNA in the chickens passing to humans.

Early on, researchers didn't think this was possible, but drug-resistant bacteria living harmlessly in the chicken, like salmonella and campylobacter, enter the human digestive system through ingested or improperly handled poultry. Once ingested, the DNA from these already resistant bacteria mutate further, creating a superbug. If a serious food-borne illness occurs, say from undercooked poultry, physicians may have to run through a series of antibiotics to find one to overcome the illness.

Before blaming the farming industry, understand that patients and physicians must take some of the blame for the problem. We create the identical scenario by not taking every last antibiotic dose the doctor prescribes and by not curbing our own antibiotic use. The Centers for Disease Control (CDC) estimated that from the mid-1980s to 2000 one-half of antibiotic prescriptions for humans were not necessary. Each time we demanded an antibiotic from our physician for mundane viral illnesses such as colds, when perhaps a little bed rest, aspirin, and fluids would do the trick, our resistance to antibiotics grew.

If your physician is stingy with his or her script writing, there is a good reason for it. The good news is antibiotic prescriptions written to treat colds and sore throats have declined, especially among children, by as much as 40%. However, physicians are still too apt to prescribe broad-spectrum antibiotics—so our own level of accountability has not yet been completely diminished.

The Antibiotic Resistance Movement

During the same time that humans popped too many antimicrobials, the feed and farm industries were even more exuberant. From 1985 to 1999 antibiotic use among chicken producers, for purposes other than illness, rose by 307% per bird, according to reports from the Union of Concerned Scientists. Until these reports, even the animal feed and veterinary industries had no idea how many antibiotics were in the farming system.

The class of antibiotics called fluoroquinolones, used in farming and human medicine, is of particular concern because these drugs are a last hope for physicians treating particularly virulent infections, including food-borne illnesses. Unfortunately, soon after fluoroquinolones were introduced into veterinary medicine in 1995 human resistance patterns began emerging. Once this cycle begins, it's impossible to stop the momentum.

Changes are afoot. In 2000 the FDA, USDA, and CDC began monitoring antibiotic use on the farm and in human medicine. A congressional bill, the Preservation of Antibiotics for Medical Treatment Act, is calling for a phaseout of eight medically important antibiotics as feed additives, as well as a requirement for drug manufacturers to report just how many antibiotics are being used and for what purpose. The FDA prefers to examine each veterinary drug and its impact on human health individually—referred to as the "bug drug" paradigm. Most recently the FDA banned the use of Baytril, a fluoroquinolone.

Many producers have already begun the slow march toward the inevitable without waiting for government rulings. In April 2006, Foster Farms, Gold Kist, Perdue, and Tyson Foods reported they had stopped using antibiotics for growth promotion, as well as significantly curbed antibiotic use for disease prevention. Tyson Foods and Foster Farms say only 1% of their flocks receive antibiotics to treat disease and none are human-grade drugs, while Perdue reports that in five years the company has resorted to using antibiotics only once to treat disease.

For years poultry associations and the animal feed industry have refused to accept their role in antibiotic resistance, citing human abuse as the primary cause. A spokesperson for the National Chicken Council used the metaphor that the "medical community sees a speck in the industry's eyes, yet they can't see the beam in their own." Richard Lobb, the outspoken spokesperson, likes to throw out a statistic that human abuse of antibiotics is as high as 90%. I looked into it—that particular study was conducted in Malaysia, where antibiotics are sold over the counter like candy. Despite Lobb's assertions, it's clear that the food system has an equal role with human medicine.

It's discouraging that, even with voluntary changes, it may not be enough to rid the food system of the resistant strains for some time. A year after Tyson and Perdue reportedly stopped using fluoroquinolones, the resistant strains were still in the meat. It may take as long as five years for these virulent strains to die off because they persist in the environment and constantly mutate to survive. In addition, since poultry processors contract with multiple suppliers, each with varying degrees of commitment to curbing antibiotic use, the resistant bacteria can spread to other meat, packaging materials, and surfaces at the processing plant—further evidence that this is not an easy problem to solve.

The conventional poultry industry is finding out what the organic side of the industry has known all along. "Animals can be raised without subtherapeutic levels of antibiotics," says Dennis Stiffler, Ph.D., executive vice president for Petaluma Poultry. "It takes a commitment to genetics, nutrition, vaccines, vitamins and minerals, and the right feed," he says. "Most of all, it requires a different level of management to anticipate the problems and manage stress among the millions of birds, which, overall, reduces illness."

Arsenic in My Chicken?

The other "A" word ruffling the poultry industry is "arsenic." Arsenic? Yes, arsenic. While arsenic is naturally occurring in our water, researchers were surprised to see it in chicken. That's troubling to hear. I remember opening my first water bill after moving to California's San Joaquin Valley. Beyond the usual fees, the bill said my tap water contained unhealthy levels of arsenic.

From 1900 through to the 1980s (when I moved in), this rich fertile ground, capable of growing the most magnificent apricots, plums, almonds, and walnuts, was laced with arsenic-containing herbicides and pesticides. The groundwater was, and still is, laden with arsenic. At the time, I paid the bill and immediately called a bottled-water company.

So how did arsenic also get into my Sunday dinner roaster? Just like water in the San Joaquin Valley, the arsenic residue in poultry is caused by human meddling. Apparently, roxarsone, a frequently used chicken feed additive, has become the drug of choice to help with weight gain and feed efficiency, and improving the color of poultry meat. For the last few years, the poultry industry maintained that use of roxarsone posed no threat to humans. Now—after as much as 73% of the poultry population has been fed more than 2 million pounds per year of the arsenic additive—this theory is suspect. The additive is also affecting arsenic levels in water. When chicken manure is applied to fields with high water tables, the roxarsone transforms into a very toxic form of arsenic that pollutes drinking water.

Typically, federal monitoring tests for arsenic in chicken livers, not meat. However, independent tests show that it, too, is tainted with arsenic—the levels vary by brand. Among 155 samples tested from grocery stores and fast-food restaurants, 55% contained detectable arsenic levels, according to the Minneapolis-based Institute for Agriculture and Trade Policy (IATP).

While none of the arsenic levels in the meat or liver were near or above the FDA's toxicity echelon (500 parts per billion in meat, 2,000 ppb in liver), the results raised suspicion that the needless additive might place consumers at risk, all in the name of fatter chickens and better meat pigment. It's not likely that you will need to call the poison center after eating chicken raised with the drug. To date there is no research about the impact on human health of eating chicken from birds fed the arsenic additive, though since we eat one-third more chicken than we did when the FDA set its toxicity limits for arsenic in poultry, you may want to seek out brands that choose not to use the drug.

It's doubtful that a warning note will be inserted into chicken packaging as was in my water bill, so of the major conventional brands which they tested, Tyson and Foster Farms had the cleanest results—no arsenic was detectable in chicken breasts for either brand; Tyson thighs were clean and Foster Farms had very low levels of 4 ppb, which could be from other sources, like water. Organic brands also tested clean, but some other conventional brands had levels as high as 22 ppb. Some fast-food menu items topped out at 44 ppb.

ANIMAL WELFARE LABELS

No Antibiotics Used, or Raised Without Antibiotics   This means just that: The chickens have never received antibiotics, from birth to slaughter, as a growth promoter or as medication. If birds are diseased, they are removed from the flock, treated, and sold as conventional chicken. Often it is impossible to treat just the sick animals, so the entire flock is treated and sold to conventional suppliers.

The claim is verified periodically by the FSIS. All certified-organic chicken may carry this label, but not all chicken with this label is organic. Some suppliers don't use organic feed but follow all the other USDA organic guidelines.

You may see other phrases like "No Subtherapeutic Antibiotics Added" and "Not Fed Antibiotics," especially on marketing materials. These are contested and not well understood because they imply the chickens were not given growth-promoting antibiotics in their feed and water but may still have received antibiotics for disease. There is currently no valid system to audit this claim, because the industry and the FDA have not set baseline levels of antibiotics for growth, disease prevention, or treatment.

USDA Organic Certified   This clearly recognizable seal is a guarantee that the chickens were raised without antibiotics or synthetic pesticides and produced with specific animal welfare guidelines.

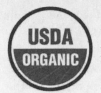

The NOP rules for organic flocks require: (1) the use of organic feed, which may not contain animal or poultry slaughter by-products; (2) the birds must have access to the outdoors, shade, shelter, exercise areas, fresh air, and direct sunlight that meet the individual needs of the species, the climate, and the environment; (3) no antibiotic use (sick hens are removed from the flock and cannot be sold as organic); (4) beak trimming is left as a farmer's decision; (5) USDA certification.

Be aware that terms like "natural" and "free-range" are popular because marketers want their chickens to appear to have the same standards as organic suppliers but without all the expense. Organic poultry suppliers often sell nonorganic lines of chicken, which are raised under similar circumstances with a few exceptions, such as nonorganic feed.

There have been attempts to dilute the definition of "organic" for poultry by producers who claim that organic feed is not always available or cost-effective. These attempts caused a great deal of alarm from organic agricultural supporters, so much so that eventually any leniency was overturned.

Biodynamic Farming This nongovernmental certified farming program declares the entire farm as sustainable and biodynamic. The rules are more stringent than those for organic food production. Biodynamic farmers adopt overall lifestyles that strive to preserve water, energy, and the surrounding natural habitat and observe farming methods that allow natural livestock behaviors. Specific to chickens: they must be outdoors as much as possible; vegetarian-fed (80% of feed must be produced on the farm); and subjected to no growth promoters, antibiotics, or practices such as debeaking and forced molting.

Cage-Free This is a misleading term used by poultry marketers. All poultry in the broiler industry are raised in cage-free barns—the equivalent of an open-floor warehouse. The number of birds and the conditions and size of the barn vary by producers; however, all chickens raised for the meat case are cage-free. So again, just like with the poultry with labels that say "no hormones," don't pay more for cage-free broilers.

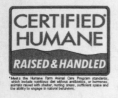

Certified Humane   Products with the Humane Farm Animal Care seal are supported by the ASPCA and the HSUS. With the support of USDA certifiers, Humane Farm Animal Care verifies that farms meet specific criteria for the humane treatment of chickens and other livestock; practices include providing clean barns with natural living space and adequate food and water and no use of antibiotics for growth promotion.

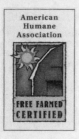

Free Farmed   The AHA developed this program to set animal welfare standards for livestock including chickens and turkeys. The chickens and turkeys are certified to indicate they live under humane conditions that allow natural behaviors, as well as receiving no antibiotics for growth promotion. Farmers are required to provide clean barns, follow safe animal husbandry guidelines, offer prompt medical treatment, and develop safe waste management systems.

Free-Range   Free-range chickens are "allowed" to go outdoors. There are no set parameters on how long this access is offered—or whether the birds actually venture out the barn door. What few realize is that broiler chickens live for only about eight weeks. It's not safe to let the chickens out of the barn for the first five of those eight, so if they do venture outdoors it's only for the last three weeks of their existence. And if they are brave enough to go outdoors, the space may be minimal or spacious, concrete or grass lined—the USDA standards for free-range are not so precise as to mandate open grassy areas, as one might imagine. In addition, all chickens raised for the broiler industry, as opposed to egg laying, are allowed to roam free in the barn. Therefore, technically all broiler chickens are cage-free, but not all chicken is free-range.

The pressure to market chickens as free-range is high because the price is higher. For instance, at Petaluma Poultry they sell two brands of broilers—Rocky Jr. and Rocky (beyond natural brand, see later) and Rosie Organic. Rocky and Rosie are free-range chickens; however, Rocky Jr. are young chickens, as the name implies. They are too young to wander out of the barn before they are sent to market—so the company doesn't sell them as free-range. A company with less ethical business practices could indeed stretch the truth in this instance; however, Petaluma honors the intent of the label.

Bird Flu and Free-Range Labels   The argument against free-range is that the environment is less controlled, which can expose the birds to a greater risk of avian disease from wild birds. Bird flu could be a major risk to the free-range label, as witnessed by worldwide concerns about avian diseases. However, free-range poultry suppliers are taking directions from the USDA and National Poultry Improvement Plan (NPIP) guidelines for biosafety by protecting birds with heavy screens and netting. It is not clear yet if the bird flu virus spreads to the United States whether the free-range label may be temporarily obsolete.

As of the summer of 2006, the bird flu virus had not spread to the United States. The rumors and myths, however, had. Here is what scientists know thus far:

1. First of all, avian flu and pandemic bird flu are not the same disease. Every year there is a certain risk for wild birds to spread avian flu to domestic poultry. The type spreading from Asia to Europe, known as the avian flu (H5N1 PAI), is of particular concern because infected wild and domestic ducks and geese show no outward symptoms (as do chickens).

2. A pandemic bird flu would be a mutation of the same virus. Pandemic bird flu occurs when the virus transforms into a genetic anomaly that can be transmitted from human to human (similar to the Spanish flu of 1918 that killed 20 to 40 million people worldwide, including 675,000 Americans). As of the summer of 2006, the only limited human-to-human transmission occurred in one Indonesian family, killing eight members. The virus did not spread to other humans outside the family.

3. Another form of transmission that worries scientists is pigs, which they suspect can harbor both the human and bird forms of the virus. It's still a hypothesis, but one that concerns investigators because if humans contracted this novel form of the virus there would be little recourse to stop the spread.

4. Despite what you may hear, free-range chicken farming has not contributed to bird flu outbreaks. If, or when, bird flu reaches this country, free-range birds may have to be contained; however, the primary source of transmission is fowl of all types that roam freely in rural neighborhoods, as is common in the two hardest-hit countries, Vietnam and Indonesia. In all but 1 case of the 127-plus human infections (since 2003), people lived and worked where poultry were allowed to roam freely and mingle with other wild bird species.

5. Thus far, there has been no transmission of avian flu from eating poultry. If chicken is properly cooked to 165 degrees Fahrenheit, the potentially infecting virus is killed.

Grass-Fed, Grass-Ranged, or Pastured Poultry   There is no USDA-approved term for 100% grass-fed poultry, nor will there be anytime soon. Unlike cows and sheep, which can live quite nicely on a diet of only grass, chickens cannot—they need a more complete diet. Chickens cannot fulfill their energy requirements from grass/forage alone, and if left to their own devices they eat bugs for protein. So while you may see marketing terms such as "100% grass-fed chickens," it's not biologically possible, nor is it likely economically feasible.

A more accurate term is "pastured poultry"; however the conditions vary significantly, according to Tom German, owner of Thankful Harvest, a beef, poultry, and egg farm that uses pastured-farming principles. A vast majority of small farmers allow their chickens to roam outdoors but supplement the bug rations with legumes, grains, fish meal, vitamins and minerals, oats, and a bit of corn. Some poultry houses are similar to conventional barns with access to the outdoors. Chicken labeled "pastured" or "grass-ranged" sometimes live in small coops that are moved frequently to fresh patches of land. Other times, because of predators, they are kept in shelters at night but allowed to roam the farmstead with no boundaries during the day.

Most often pastured poultry is sold at farmers' markets and small health-food stores, where consumers and store owners have direct access to the farmer. German recommends that consumers ask questions and "listen carefully to the answers for clues about what the operation is like." He admits this is complicated, but without monitoring, the responsibility lies with the consumer.

Hormone-Free   As you read earlier, this is a misnomer. All poultry are raised without the use of added hormones. Also, remember that all animal products contain naturally occurring hormones, so nothing red-blooded is ever really hormone-free.

Natural   The USDA definition means the chicken has been "minimally processed and contains no artificial flavoring, colors, chemical preservatives, artificial, or synthetic ingredients." It does not have anything to do with how the chickens were raised. In addition, any chicken labeled as "natural," according to the USDA definition, cannot contain any additives, so don't pay more for a brand that says "no additives or preservatives."

Beyond Natural   The health-food store definition of "natural" forbids the use of antibiotics, pesticides, or animal by-products in feed. A brand may meet the store's qualifying terms for "natural" but not be certified organic. Usually the primary difference between these brands of natural poultry and organic is the feed, which is not organic, and the lack of a certifying agency.

Stores like Wild Oats and Whole Foods use a definition of "natural" that exceeds the USDA's. Suppliers sign affidavits that state the chicken was raised in humane conditions and not raised with antibiotics, pesticides, and animal by-products. In addition, each supplier must show a paperwork trail verifying that all standards are met on a continual basis. Health-food stores usually carry a range of chicken brands that meet the strict definition of "natural" as well as "certified organic."

Many of the brands in health-food stores are venturing into mass market distribution channels. They may sit side by side with conventional brands that use the USDA watered-down definition of "natural"; you'll have to read the fine print to see the nuances.

Vegetarian-Fed   As a stand-alone label, "vegetarian-fed" doesn't have anything to do with antibiotic use. Call the producer directly if you are concerned about antibiotics, because this label doesn't necessarily mean no antibiotics were administered. Chicken skin color ranges from cream to yellow because of the type of feed—wheat, white or yellow corn. For the buyer, it's a matter of taste and preference—not quality, value, or tenderness.

PROCESSING LABELS

USDA Poultry Grading and Types   These are verified by the FSIS, USDA, and individual state inspectors. The FSIS inspects all interstate, imported, and exported poultry. In-state inspection services must be at least equal to FSIS programs.

Grade A is the highest-quality chicken grade and the primary grade sold at grocery stores. This label is voluntary—twenty-six states use USDA inspectors; the remaining have their own meat and poultry grading inspection systems that meet USDA standards.

When you see this symbol, the poultry is free of defects such as bruises, discolorations, and feathers. Bone-in products have no broken bones; skin is free of tears and has a consistent layer of fat under the skin. Whole chickens must be meaty and fully fleshed. The grade shield is on all chilled, frozen, and ready-to-cook chicken roasts and parts. There are no grades for necks, wings, giblets, or ground poultry. Grades B and C are lower poultry grades, usually for processed products.

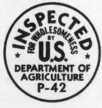

This is a mandatory federal label that guarantees inspections for safety, sanitation, and labeling standards. After years of lax oversight, the FDA and FSIS developed a step-by-step system to improve the safety of meat and poultry during production and distribution (called the Hazard Analysis and Critical Control Points, HACCP, implemented in

2000). Unlike the USDA label, which is a measure of quality, this label ensures that certain minimum safety standards have been met.

Salmonella rates were at their lowest in 2000 at 9%; however, by 2005 the rates jumped back up to 16%. In July 2006, a consumer advocacy group released the names of poultry processors whose plants had failed federal standards for salmonella. Food & Water Watch obtained the numbers from the USDA; it was the first ever release of such information by the agency. Food & Water is calling for the USDA to ask federal regulators to pass legislation that requires HACCP standards to be enforceable and require the posting of the results for each plant on the Internet (the USDA plans to post the collective results each quarter). Overall, the results released to Food & Water showed the salmonella rates for poultry dropped to 12% in the first quarter of 2006, a 4% improvement from 2005.

Freshness Dates and Packing Codes   Federal law doesn't require product dating for poultry, but grocers prefer the dates to help manage inventory. Some are safety related; others have more to do with quality.

Open Dating uses a calendar date, rather than a code date, to remind the store how long to sell the product and helps you know when a product might be past its prime. Here are the different types:

> **Sell-By Date** is a voluntary label that tells the store how long the product can be sold. It's usually about seven to ten days from the time the chickens were slaughtered. For optimum safety, cook or freeze raw chicken within one or two days of purchase; unopened precooked chicken may hold for three to four days.

> **The Best-If-Used-Before Date** is a measure of quality, not safety.

> **The Use-By Date** is set by the manufacturer as the best time to cook or freeze the product. It's best not to exceed this date for raw or precooked chicken.

Closed or Coded Dates are the packing numbers and internal dating codes used by the manufacturers. There is no standardized system for closed dates; however, this number is an important tracking tool if you ever get sick. Here is how Tyson uses closed dates. Example: 227 3 PLA 01 14

227 is the Julian Date for August 15.

3 is the year, 2003.

PLA is the Tyson Plant.

01 is the production line.

14 is 1400, military time for 2:00 P.M., the hour of production.

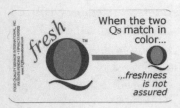

FRESHNESS LABELS

This label came from the same technology used in airports for homeland security. Instead of detecting explosives, these highly sensitive sensors identify when the chicken is spoiled by changing the label color. The color change sends out a message to the shopper to leave this package in the case. The labels, called FreshQ, change from a fresh tangerine color to gray when the meat is spoiled. Look for them on chicken, beef, and pork.

Enhanced Chicken Producers inject or marinade poultry with broth, water, salt, or phosphates, increasing the weight by as much as 15%. Poultry processing involves volumes and volumes of water to clean and adequately chill the chicken. As a result, a small percentage of water clings to the chicken, adding negligible weight. This is different from enhanced chicken.

Fresh Chicken As much as I would like to put this label in the questionable category, the rules regarding fresh chicken are there to prevent the spread of bacteria. A chicken can be chilled to between twenty-six to thirty-two degrees Fahrenheit, hard enough to break your kitchen window, but still be called fresh. The rule was adopted to allow for safe transport of chicken, since food-borne bacteria thrive at temperatures approaching forty degrees. Poultry held at temperatures between zero and twenty-four degrees has no specific labeling; anything below zero degrees is considered truly frozen.

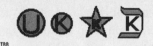

KOSHER POULTRY CERTIFICATION

Kosher certification is represented most often by either a *U* or *K*, enclosed in a circle, star, or other graphic—there are as many as 600 symbols to designate kosher (most are protected trademarks). Kosher-certified food meets specific dietary rules as defined by Jewish law and is inspected by independent agencies that monitor foods for compliance.

Ritual slaughter is known as *shechitah*; the person who performs the slaughter is called a *schochet*. The method of slaughter is a quick, deep stroke across the throat with a sharp blade, which is designed to be painless and humane and cause unconsciousness within two seconds. This method ensures rapid, complete draining of the blood, which is necessary to render the meat kosher. The meat is also carefully examined to make certain that no blood, sciatic nerves, blood vessels, or *chelev* (a type of fat that surrounds vital organs and the liver) is present. The *shochet* is not just a butcher—he should be pious and well trained in Jewish law, particularly as it relates to Jewish food laws (kashruth). In smaller venues, the rabbi and the *shochet* are often the same person. Kosher certification of poultry has attracted attention of non-Jews because of the humane slaughtering methods and careful inspection practices.

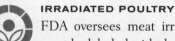

IRRADIATED POULTRY

FDA oversees meat irradiation and all irradiated poultry must be labeled with the radura symbol. Irradiation reduces most, but not all, salmonella levels in chicken by either electron accelerators, X-ray generators, or radionuclides, a radioactive material that gives off ionizing gamma rays.

The Center for Consumer Research, a pro-irradiation group, says that the taste, texture, and color of chicken are not affected by low-level irradiation. However, food tasters report that irradiated chicken is tougher, the taste is a bit off, and the chicken has an unnerving red hue. To counter the ill-perceived color and flavor changes, food scientists use either a synthetic substance called TBHQ or natural extracts from rosemary and grape seeds.

Florida is the only state with notable marketing and sales for irradiated chicken. Critics are fearful that irradiation is an excuse to ignore farming conditions that lead to food-borne illnesses. Proponents of irradiation agree that irradiation shouldn't preclude clean farming practices, only augment them.

Irradiation doesn't kill all the bacteria—improper storing, handling, and cooking techniques can still open the door for food-borne illnesses. In addition, food irradiation does not kill botulism, ever, so be aware of spoiled precooked foods. Irradiation also slightly reduces levels of vitamins A, C, E, and K and thiamine, although researchers advise that unless your diet is based mostly on irradiated products there is little risk of a deficiency.

SAFE HANDLING AND COOKING INSTRUCTION LABEL

Food-borne bacteria, such as campylobacter, can survive refrigeration, which means there are multiple opportunities for the bacteria to spread during processing, transportation to the store, and in your grocery cart. In addition, salmonella percentages for broilers are squirrelly. From 2002 to 2004 they crept up from 11.5% to 13.5%, and in 2005 they spiked to 16.3%. For ground poultry it's even higher. In 2005 32.4% of ground chicken and 23.2% of ground turkey tested positive, which was also a slight increase from previous years. This means that you should always use the plastic bags at the meat counter to prevent leaky chicken packages from contaminating your entire grocery purchase and your hands.

The bacteria in chicken thrive prolifically when the temperature climbs above forty degrees. So it's also best to purchase chicken last when shopping and avoid making any last-minute errands on the way home. In a car with ninety-degree heat, chicken will begin to spoil within one hour; at room temperature, two hours.

At home, store the chicken in the refrigerator at forty degrees or less for up to two days depending on the sell-by or use-by date. Chicken can be frozen at zero degrees for an indefinite amount of time, as long as there is no change in temperature. However, after about two to three months freezer burn will set in, affecting the taste and texture.

Make certain the internal temperature of chicken breasts reaches 165 degrees. The minimum oven temperature for cooking poultry is 325 degrees. Do not partially cook chicken and refrigerate it for later use; you'll only invite trouble for dinner.

Many recipes call for rinsing chicken before cooking; the USDA says this isn't good advice, since the bacteria can spread more easily to other areas of the kitchen. When preparing a chicken recipe, premeasure all the other ingredients and have them on hand before you touch the chicken. This will prevent you from opening cupboards and drawers, which can easily spread bacteria around the kitchen. Reserve a separate cutting board for chicken and another for vegetables. Wash your hands often with soap and warm water when handling raw chicken, as well as all utensils, plates, countertops, and cutting boards.

Bottom Line

The argument as to who is responsible for antibiotic resistance, and to what effect, is an old one that should be laid to rest. In all the disagreement, there is one question: who is better served by antibiotics, 290 million Americans or 8 billion chickens a year? For a parent comforting a child with a food-borne illness or a sister holding the hand of an elderly brother dying from pneumonia, the cost of human health and life is immeasurable and certainly worth more than a few cents more per pound for safer food.

I applaud the poultry suppliers that have stopped using human-grade antibiotics. Now perhaps other major suppliers will make similar changes, if not only for their customers also for their employees and local community. Studies show that regions in the South, where most broiler chickens are raised, have extraordinary levels of antibiotic resistance.

For years the persistent challenge to reducing antibiotic use was always money and the threat that higher prices will ensue if human-grade antibiotics are banned. As a consumer who is fairly price conscious, I haven't noticed any big price hikes since Foster Farms, Tyson, and Purdue began curbing antibiotic use.

At the low end, the World Health Organization estimated a *zero* price hike if human-grade antibiotics were prohibited. At the most, the National Research Council predicted consumers might pay one to three cents more per pound for chicken and two to three cents more per pound for turkey raised with fewer antibiotics. That's not much considering the estimated health cost to society for resistance to one single commonly prescribed antibiotic, amoxicillin, is $225 million per year and overall cost for all antibiotic resistance is $4 to $5 billion to U.S. society and individuals yearly.

As with many changes, the ultimate solutions lie outside Capitol Hill, beyond the boardrooms of veterinary drug companies, and far from the demands of corporate accountants. Researchers unencumbered by such influence say the laboratory and the farm hold the answers and the consumer dollar holds the power. As the argument for excessive antibiotics is shot down by research showing that farm-use antibiotics do place humans most at risk, it is indeed time for new ideas that don't sacrifice human safety for the same old chicken recipe.

CHAPTER 4

The Hard-Boiled Facts About Egg Labels

Ruffled Feathers

When I walked into the barn at Hillside Egg Farm in Niwot, Colorado, I mentally prepared for the stench. Climbing the flight of stairs to the henhouse, I couldn't hold my breath any longer and inhaled. I waited for the eye-watering, throat-stinging ammonia smell—nothing happened.

The day turned out to be a lesson in disbelief. The barn didn't smell and the egg farmer and egg company CEO leading me upstairs didn't fit my expectations. When he isn't farming, Dave Turunjian is an accountant, and the CEO of Nest Fresh Eggs, Cyd Szymanski, looks more like a suburban soccer mom than the owner of chicken farms.

We talked while standing in the middle of the henhouse. Thousands of white-feathered birds, with rose-colored combs, milled around our ankles. I haven't been this close to chickens since I was fifteen, when on a visit to my dad's farm he pointed to the chicken coop, handed me a bucket of feed, and reminded me to take a baseball bat to fend off the roosters.

Even Szymanski is leery from being pecked at as a child, but this wasn't bad at all. The hens are free to roam on a plastic floor permeated with holes for the feathers and manure to fall through. Henhouses, lined with gray Astroturf (the hens like gray better than green, Szymanski tells me), split the barn into two sections. A conveyor belt catches the eggs and moves them into the packing house. It's all very clean and tidy.

When Turunjian agreed to supply eggs for Szymanski's company he had to convert his caged operations to cage-free. To do so, he needed to add a barn and cut his bird population down from 30,000 to 13,000 hens. Harder yet, he had to convince Boulder County that the expansion wouldn't interfere with the local community. By local community, he means $3 million 10,000-square-foot homes that sit a stone's throw from the farm—it's a little like Green Acres meets the Hiltons.

To gain their approval, Turunjian did the unthinkable. He invited some of the wealthiest and most pampered citizens of the community to stand, just as I did, in the barn and take a whiff. They inhaled and approved the permit. Eight years later there have been no complaints about offensive odors from neighbors.

Perhaps it is Szymanski's gumption to redefine her family's way of life that inspired Turunjian to go to the trouble. Szymanski grew up in Missouri, where the family business is eggs. It's also where she was told the male-dominated caged-egg industry was no place for a woman. Her family founded MOARK, one of the largest traditional egg companies in the nation, which sells eggs under the Land O Lakes brand.

Szymanski detoured away from the family biz for a while, but the pull to do what she had done her whole life—raise laying hens for eggs—was too great. With the help of her brother and her father, who pulled up Missouri stakes, she started an egg business with a new set of rules—no cages, only vegetarian diets, and no antibiotics. Szymanski admits her rationale in 1990 was a blend of family defiance and a woman's scorn.

Sixteen years later, her hunch to go her own way has gained back some long-lost relatives. Mark and May Belle Adams, Szymanski's aunt and uncle, see value in their niece's methods. May Belle and Mark went head to head with the family business by joining citizens in Neosha, Missouri, to fight a permit request for MOARK to expand production from 2.5 to 5 million hens by building new, modern egg houses. Citizens collected 3,500 signatures to fight the expansion, citing complaints ranging from soil contamination to an unpleasant layer of ammonia fumes that hangs over the region, referred to as "MOARK mornings." No one wanted the plant shut down, just cleaned up before any notions of expansion were decided.

For MOARK officials the modernization process was moving along well until the company was cited for animal abuse—a passerby on the way to his son's soccer game (with a video camera in the car) filmed workers throwing live MOARK hens for disposal into a tractor trailer. As restitution, MOARK agreed to finance a local humane society with a $100,000 donation and to overhaul its euthanasia procedures for spent hens in exchange for animal cruelty charges being dropped.

Citizens were hopeful that this coincidental predicament would help stall the expansion plans; however, in the fall of 2005 the Missouri Department of Natural Resources approved the development. "I thought that because I was family I could make a difference," said May Belle. "It didn't work." According to MOARK's press release, the new facilities are so top-of-the-line that citizens like the Adamses will be free of the frequent odor problem. The traditional manure pits that caused the ever-familiar stench will remove waste immediately on belts that carry it away for disposal. Even with the modern equipment, there is no way to predict whether the transition will go as well as Turunjian's Hillside Egg Farm expansion. And you thought your family holidays were stressful. . . .

Who Is Minding the Henhouse?

It's lucky for the industry that eggs are sold by the dozen, because egg cartons are covered with more labels than any other food packaging. No other food sector has used labels to address such a wide swath of consumer and industry issues, including animal welfare, food-borne illnesses, and nutritional concerns. The ten-by-three-inch carton is valuable real-estate space for words like "free-range," "free-roaming," "vegetarian fed," and "cage-free" and nutrient claims for vitamin E and omega-3s. Even eggshells may be billboards, with sell-by dates or company logos stamped on each egg. Egg labels are about what the marketers "want" us to believe.

Animal welfare claims, such as free-range, are a "mixed bag," says Deanna Baldwin, Maryland state egg inspector and member of the National Egg Regulatory Officials (NERO), an agency that tracks state egg laws and practices. She says that in her state inspection agents monitor animal welfare claims through a word-of-mouth net-work, citing any violations as they occur. However, unless there are federal rules and enough officials to enforce them, state inspectors can't do much more. This leaves marketers free to use just the right terms that will draw consumers to their products, regardless of whether the hens are raised with progressive farming practices or not.

The chasm of interpretation for animal-welfare claims for hens is largely a result of a fractional oversight process that varies from agency to agency, state to state, and processor to processor. Within the government sector, shell eggs are under the purview of the FDA; however, the inspection process, labeling, and marketing are parsed out to the USDA's FSIS and Agricultural Marketing Service.

The USDA inspects eggs and applies its agency's rules for labeling claims, but USDA inspections are voluntary. American hens lay more than 72 billion eggs per year; the USDA inspects about one-third of them. The remaining 52 billion eggs are overseen by individual state inspection offices, each with their own sets of standards for animal welfare labeling claims and inspections.

There seem to be no shortages of vibrant casts of characters that set up undercover investigations against suspect farms. Animal wel-fare groups constantly accuse egg farms of nurturing the bottom line instead of healthy flocks. Activists further use the hens' plight to jump-start interest in vegan lifestyles. Standing on the sidelines, often absorbing contradictory information, are egg consumers, who most likely have never even set foot on a chicken farm.

Food marketers play on consumer confusion by bringing atten-tion to single issues or "motivators," said Katherine DiMatteo, the former executive director of the Organic Trade Association, in Greenfield, Massachusetts. If you take into account each individual health, safety, and animal welfare issue the egg industry has dealt with since the late 1980s, you'll find a label perfectly matched to a specific egg-farming practice that has been under the microscope—"cage-free" addresses overcrowding, "vegetarian-fed hens" is the term for no animal by-products in feed, "free-range" implies a pristine pas-tured setting, and "natural" is perceived by consumers as meaning antibiotic- or pesticide-free. Look closer at the actual definition and you will see that some terms fall short of matching our city-folk-accepted wisdom.

The best documented example of profiting from questionable labeling came when a Chicago-based nonprofit group, Food Animal Concern Trust (FACT), studied whether eggs could be produced in a humane manner and still be profitable, a claim refuted by conven tional egg producers. To fund the research, FACT marketed humanely produced eggs under the NEST EGGS label and sold them at a premium price, said Kathy Seuss, farm program and public education manager. The higher margins were too good for some nearby egg farmers to resist, according to Seuss. Soon after NEST EGGS reached the marketplace, competitors labeled their eggs with similar wording and sold their eggs a lower price than FACT's cost of production, without necessarily making any changes in production practices. For FACT, they didn't have to worry about competitive pressure to stay afloat; however, for actual egg producers such actions could mean financial ruin.

Poor Sales and Sickness Prompt Lifestyle Change for Hens

If one peels away the layers of concern from each of the groups, there is a kernel of truth within each of their arguments. Yes, for better health, all Americans should eat more vegetables and fewer animal products. Yes, farming practices should require the humane treatment of hens, for their health as well as ours. And yes, farming is big business, which means there is a constant balancing act between shareholders, the farmers, and the price the market will support.

But in the end, it was human illness from eggs infected with a destructive pathogen that brought the fractious parties together. In the latter half of the 1990s, the treatment of hens was no longer perceived as just a health issue for fowl but also one for humans. The discovery of a new bacterium, living inside the chicken and the egg, changed people's minds. Previously most strains could be managed by washing eggs and cleaning out the barn, but this new bug, *Salmonella enterica* (SE), lived inside the chicken and transferred to the egg.

The sheer volume of complaints by Consumers Union and the Center for Science in the Public Interest, as well as the General Accounting Office and CDC, finally caught the interest of the FDA. "Conditions in the country's egg farms aren't just bad news for the chickens. They are serious environmental and health concerns for people as well," reported Consumers Union in their eco-label report on eggs.

Testimonies and reports on egg safety connected the dots and scientifically linked 2.3 million SE-contaminated eggs per year to hundreds of thousands of illnesses. In 1999, human illness from SE cost Americans from $.5 to $2.3 billion in medical care and lost productivity due to food-borne infections. The science, not reports from activists, illustrates that salmonella rates had risen because of a lack of guidelines for egg refrigeration and basic food safety standards.

The reports changed the tide of concern. Consumers didn't have to be card-carrying members of an animal rights group to care about the welfare of American hens, because no longer was the desperate condition of egg farms solely an animal welfare issue. These unhealthy living conditions translated into human health concerns directly related to questionable farming practices and poorly designed food safety regulations.

The egg industry responded to the criticism with its own statistical calculations—1 egg per 20,000 could be contaminated with SE, meaning the average consumer would encounter a contaminated egg only once in eighty-four years. One critic said shoppers had a better chance of being in a car accident on the way to the store to buy the eggs than getting sick from eating eggs.

In truth, no one was really sure how many people actually died or became ill from SE, since most illnesses went unreported, because the symptoms develop as soon as eight hours or as far away as three days from ingestion, when the infecting egg or food is far from memory. No matter how the egg industry ran the numbers, the transmission of SE increased eightfold from 1976 to 1995. By 2004, the USDA and the FSIS had enough sound data to assess just how many eggs contained SE and how many illnesses might result. According to the data, 350,000 illnesses per year are predicted from SE in shell eggs.

Years of reactionary measures designed to produce eggs in the easiest and least expensive way possible all contributed to the increased SE pathogens in eggs. The rationale of profit at any cost no longer held true when egg sales declined, reaching an all-time low in the early 1990s. The industry got the message and began cleaning up the barn and their image. In August 1998, President Clinton's administration established the President's Council on Food Safety to protect Americans against food-borne illnesses. The resulting Egg Safety Task Force subcommittee began an action plan to eliminate SE bacteria in eggs.

It has taken since 1998 for the language in the Shell Egg Safety Action Plan program to be finalized, which will require egg farms with 3,000 or more laying hens to include some commonsense measures like mandatory pest and rodent control, disinfection of poultry houses, SE lab testing, and egg refrigeration. In addition, the feed and birds that enter the farm will be certified as free of SE by NPIP suppliers.

The changes could prompt major declines in SE—practices as simple and intuitive as refrigerating eggs within twelve hours of lay through to packaging and shipping could reduce the number of human illnesses by 273,000 per year. The final USDA rules for the Egg Safety Task Force will be approved in 2006–2007. The hope is that SE outbreaks will decline by at least half by 2010.

Is There a Fox in the Henhouse of Self-Regulation?

The egg industry's first major attempt to regulate itself for animal welfare issues was met with a quirk of fate that didn't help their cause. In 2002, the United Egg Producers (UEP), the egg industry's trade association for animal welfare and government lobbying, decided that instead of constantly barring the barn door to consumer concerns about the plight of its egg-laying hens they, too, would develop a voluntary animal welfare label, the "Animal Care Certified" label.

To display the labels, farms had to agree to a set of guidelines that addressed issues such as cleanliness, water and feed requirements, cage space allowance, beak trimming, and induced molting. UEP, the industry's largest trade organization, believed that the parameters adequately addressed animal welfare issues for egg-laying hens.

Animal welfare groups took interest in the Animal Care Certified label, hoping that it would prompt changes. Upon review, critics said it wasn't enough—the rules still tipped greatly in favor of the egg industry because it upped battery cage space (wire cages) by only a few inches, rather than banning them outright, and the certification still allowed practices the animal welfare groups despised, like induced molting (by withholding feed) and beak trimming with no anesthesia. "When they see the Animal Care Certified logo on an egg carton, most consumers don't think the birds laying those eggs live in cages so tight they can't even flap their wings," said Paul Shapiro, campaign director for Compassion Over Killing (COK), an animal welfare and vegetarian lifestyle nonprofit group.

Groups like COK wanted the egg industry to turn itself inside out. UEP responded by saying that their program was science based and relied on the advice of veterinary exports and scientists and, for the time being, the standards would remain as they were designed in order to maintain current supplies without price spikes, adding that any further changes would be phased in over time.

In 2004, COK secretly taped the conditions of a Maryland farm using the Animal Care Certified logo. COK alleged the hens were caught between bars, unable to get to food or water, and dead birds were left in various stages of decay throughout the barn. The conditions caught on tape raised questions as to whether the definition of "humane treatment" was lost only on this particular farm or if these conditions were industrywide.

The video may have raised doubts as to whether the egg industry was capable of regulating itself. In all fairness, one had to consider the source of the tape with some skepticism, as COK promotes animal welfare rights *and* vegan lifestyles.

COK's covert operation caught the attention of the Better Business Bureau's National Advertising Division and called into question whether the label was misleading to consumers. After reviewing statements from both UEP and COK, the advertising division advised the egg trade association to discontinue the label because "the animal care message is likely to mislead consumers for an issue that may be important to their purchasing decision."

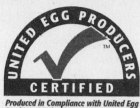

Produced in Compliance with United Egg
Producers' Animal Husbandry Guidelines
www.uepcertified.com

In October 2005, the trade group changed the text of its Animal Care Certified logo to say "United Egg Producers Certified" and, in smaller type, "Produced in Compliance with United Egg Producers' Animal Husbandry Guidelines." The new labeling guidelines made one concession: the practice of induced molting by withholding feed would be banned. Was this enough for COK? Let's start with a lesson in egg farming, and then you can decide.

Egg Farming 101

Animal welfare groups like COK have penned terms like "debeaking," "forced molting," and "battery cages" to draw attention to the condition of American egg farms. Most consumers have little understanding about what these terms really mean. The following are explanations of each practice and the dividing opinions, where much of the squabble lies. The first term is according to the animal welfare rights groups; the second is preferred by the farming industry:

DEBEAKING/BEAK TRIMMING
"Debeaking" is the inflammatory word for beak trimming because it implies that hen's beaks are completely removed, which is not the case no matter how the hens are raised. Although you may see Web sites with unsightly photos of hens with scorched beaks, beak trimming is the preferred and most widely used method. A few days after birth, the chicks' beaks are snipped to remove a sharp knob and hook on the end of each beak.

You've heard the expression "pecking order." This is exactly how chickens decide who is dominant; they peck at one another—it's the equivalent of alpha-dog behavior. To avoid the bloodletting, beak trimming is common. In fact, the practice is so widespread that even some animal rights activist groups have backpedaled and are asking that beak trimming be done with anesthesia but not banned outright. The only certified farming practice that prohibits beak trimming is biodynamic farming. Organic certification allows the farmer to decide on a case-by-case basis whether to trim beaks.

FORCED MOLTING/INDUCED MOLTING

The average hen lays an egg every twenty-seven hours and does so for about eighteen months before it is sent to slaughter for processed foods, such as frozen dinners and chicken nuggets. As the hens age, their productivity declines, so to induce a few more laying cycles farmers use a method called induced molting—animal rights groups call it "forced molting." Molting is a normal occurrence when hens' hormone levels decline, appetite drops, and feathers fall out—it's somewhat like a four-month perimenopause for hens. When this un-avoidable reproductive metamorphosis is over, the hens lay eggs for a few more cycles. To speed this cycle up by about two months and make the hens molt all at the same time, farmers can induce the molt by reducing feed nutrients, altering barn lighting to disrupt the hens' sleep cycle, and withholding feed, a practice animal rights groups call starvation.

No matter what it is called, the practice of withholding feed to in-duce molting has been greatly criticized by veterinarians as well as ac-tivists as inhumane. Now that the new UEP certification policy forbids withholding food, farmers will instead use low-nutrient diets to induce molting. From a health perspective, there are studies showing that in-duced molting from withdrawing feed actually increases the level of salmonella infection in the hens and eggs—UEP's decision to forbid this practice, as well as the newly implemented plans of the Egg Safety Task Force, will, I hope, reduce human salmonella exposure.

BATTERY CAGES/CAGES

This is perhaps the most touchy subject in egg farming. As much as 90% of the egg industry worldwide uses wire cages to house hens. In the United States, about 90% of the egg industry is UEP certified, so this group gets the most heat for using cages. The UEP certification has increased cage space from forty-eight to sixty-seven inches; compliance must be achieved by 2008. The association may increase cage space even more in the future. The trade association still stands firmly behind the use of cages because they believe cages prevent aggressive behavior and allow for better farm management, which keeps egg prices within an affordable price range. Above all, UEP says it bases its decisions on science, not emotions.

Naturally these points are disputed by cage-free egg producers and activists who say open barns reduce stress and that cages cause leg injuries and even death, as well as prohibiting natural behaviors like preening, scratching, and nesting. The E.U. is often held up as the model of cage-free eggs, because battery cages will be banned by 2012. This does not mean that that European egg producers won't use confinement, but the cages will be larger and more refined. Enriched cages have a nest, a litter for pecking and scratching, and perch space—a hen penthouse of sorts.

Wire cages remain a thorny reality of this country's egg-farming system and there is no hint that American birds will move to a better neighborhood of enriched cages anytime soon. It's interesting to note than many UEP-certified farms raise both cage-free and caged hens for eggs, both with wide-ranging price points. UEP says the hens are raised under identical conditions with the exception of cages. In the future, UEP is planning to develop cage-free guidelines that determine the best space parameters for cage-free barns.

The trend for producers to market both caged and cage-free hens has prompted new marketing slogans that tout "no cages, ever." I'm not sure the egg carton has room for any more labels; however, the issue has become one of consumer choice—which, for me, is always a good thing.

To date, under very public pressure from groups like COK, Trader Joe's in the United States has converted its private label brands to cage-free. Eggs sold at many chains, including Whole Foods, Wild Oats, Earth Fare, and Jimbo's . . . Naturally! are completely cage-free. Even Google, headquartered in Mountain View, California, has agreed to buy its 300,000 eggs a year and 7,000 pounds of liquid egg products from cage-free suppliers. Last and certainly not least, Wal-Mart stores in the U.K. have agreed to switch the store brand to cage-free before the 2012 deadline—no such changes have occurred as of this writing at stateside Wal-Marts; stay tuned.

Egg Labeling

Since the FDA's primary concern is egg safety, not animal welfare, it may take some time to rein in wayward animal welfare claims on egg cartons. Until that time comes, if you are a shopper who takes a genuine interest in animal welfare claims, buy eggs from a certified farm with careful oversight; otherwise you might not get what you think you are paying for. If you are a shopper who likes to prioritize your concerns rather than buy into the entire package, then read on.

FOOD SAFETY AND INSPECTION LABELS

All labels within this category are certified by a U.S. government agency or a nongovernmental third party. Unless outright fraud is a factor, you can be assured that these labels and their respective farming practices are monitored regularly.

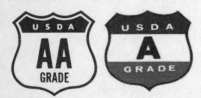

USDA Egg Grading and Size Hold an egg to a bright light in a dark room and you'll see lines and specks marking the shell, a cloudy-white albumen surrounding the yolk, and a small pocket, or the air cell, at the top of the egg. Each of these factors determines whether an egg will be graded AA, A, or B, in descending order. For instance, an AA egg will have a one-eighth-inch air cell equaling the size of a dime and a thick egg white.

About 70% of eggs are graded by state agencies, which follow USDA grading guidelines; the remaining eggs are inspected by the USDA, as indicated by the USDA crest on cartons. The average eye can't see a difference between AA and A eggs, and grade B eggs are mostly prebroken and sent to bakeries, food-service operations, and pasteurization plants.

Egg Quality   In addition to grading eggs, the USDA monitors egg farms (not just contracted farms) for eggshell quality, making certain that cracked, leaky, bloody, or dirty eggs don't get into the food supply. Occasionally you may find blood spots in eggs; this does not mean the egg is unsafe. It means one or more small blood vessels in the yolk ruptured at the time of ovulation. If you purchase eggs from small farms you may see more bloody spots than in USDA-inspected eggs because not all small farms that sell directly to consumers check for blood spots.

Most recipes, especially in baking, call for large eggs, but egg sizes range from small, medium, large, and extra-large to jumbo. To substitute another size, the following equivalents work:

Large	Jumbo	Extra-Large	Medium	Small
1	1	1	1	1
2	2	2	2	3
3	2	3	3	4
4	3	4	5	5
5	4	4	6	7
6	5	5	7	8

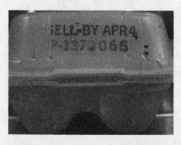

Freshness Dates and Packing Codes
If you take eggs out of the carton and store them in an open plastic egg holder in your refrigerator, reconsider. You should keep the eggs in the cardboard carton. Egg inspectors say each time you open the refrigerator the eggs are prone to temperature fluctuations, which can help SE cells multiply to unhealthy levels.

In addition, all USDA-inspected eggs require packing dates and plant numbers. If by chance you get sick from the eggs or the quality is not up to par, these numbers are traceable digits to identify the source, should you want to take action. Here's an explanation of all those dates and numbers:

Expiration dates and sell-by dates are dates that extend no later than thirty days from the day the eggs were packed. On average, eggs will last three weeks from these dates.

Use-by, use-before, and best-before dates are dates that indicate the expected length of time the eggs maintain their quality when stored in ideal conditions, or about forty-five days from the packing date. These dates are optional for USDA-inspected eggs.

Plant numbers are preceded by a *P*, as in P-1379, as seen in the carton photo shown on previous page. Some state laws require a state's abbreviation with the plant number.

Packing dates are the day of the year the eggs were processed and placed into the cartons. Ideally, this is within one week of egg laying, but it can take longer for the eggs to get from the farm to the packing plant—so buy eggs with the most recent date available. Packing dates are expressed as on the Julian calendar, which assigns a number to each day of the year—001 for January 1 and 365 for December 31. For instance, the carton shown previously says "066," which means March 7, 2005.

If for some reason you aren't certain if the egg is fresh, crack it open. Egg white color is a good indicator of the egg's age and safety—a cloudy white means it's very fresh; clear whites are from older but still safe eggs, and pinkish egg whites mean the egg is spoiled. Blood specks in egg yolks are safe, although unappealing.

Regardless of best-by, sell-by, or any other date on the label, buy clean and uncracked eggs. If you buy them from a grocery store, don't wash them. The eggs are washed, sanitized, and coated with a tasteless mineral oil that protects the shell. Refrigerate them right away and don't keep them at room temperature for more than two hours. Wash your hands, utensils, equipment, and work areas with hot, soapy water before and after contact with eggs.

Pasteurized   Pasteurized shell eggs are heated to a very high temperature for a second or less to reduce salmonella contamination. All pre-broken eggs sold as a liquid in cartons are pasteurized. Pasteurization will kill most, but not all, SE bacteria, and there is still a possibility that the SE can return. It is estimated that liquid pasteurized eggs cause 50,000 illnesses a year.

The pasteurization process and its respective machinery are monitored by the Food Safety Inspection Agency and approved by the FDA. To date, there are only a few plants that pasteurize shell eggs. Often pasteurized-egg cartons are sealed in plastic to prevent repacking broken eggs. Pasteurized eggs are useful for recipes that call for raw eggs, such as meringues, ice creams, and salad dressings.

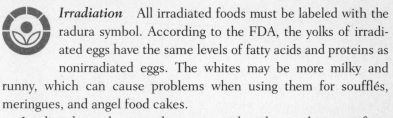 *Irradiation*   All irradiated foods must be labeled with the radura symbol. According to the FDA, the yolks of irradiated eggs have the same levels of fatty acids and proteins as nonirradiated eggs. The whites may be more milky and runny, which can cause problems when using them for soufflés, meringues, and angel food cakes.

Irradiated eggs have not been met with widespread interest from consumers and, therefore, are not commonly sold in stores. Critics of the poor conditions at egg farms and packing plants say that neither irradiation nor pasteurization is an acceptable substitute for cleaning up unsanitary farms.

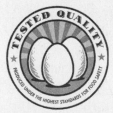 *Egg Quality Assurance Programs (EQAP)*   If you buy eggs with this seal in Pennsylvania, consider yourself lucky. The state adopted a comprehensive egg safety program, the Pennsylvania Egg Quality Assurance Program (PEQAP), long before the FDA ever got around to a similar program. There are now at least fifteen states with state- or industry-led programs: Pennsylvania, Connecticut, California, South Carolina, Maryland, Ohio, Michigan, Utah, New York, Alabama, Louisiana, Indiana, Oregon, Florida, and Georgia. When the

federal egg safety laws go into effect, they will fundamentally mimic these programs.

CERTIFIED ANIMAL WELFARE LABELS

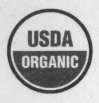

USDA Organic   Since October 2002 organic eggs have had a recognizable USDA seal that guarantees the laying hens were raised without antibiotics or pesticides and produced within specific animal welfare guidelines. Be aware, though, that terms like "natural," "free-range," and "cage-free" are popular because marketers want their eggs to appear to have the same quality controls as organic suppliers.

The NOP rules for organic flocks require: (1) the use of organic feed, which may not contain animal or poultry slaughter by-products, but there are no restrictions for fish meal; (2) access to the outdoors for the birds (they may be temporarily confined only for reasons of health, safety, or the animal's stage of production or to protect soil or water quality); (3) barn lighting no longer than the longest day of the year; (4) no antibiotic use (sick hens are removed from the flock and the eggs cannot be sold as organic); (5) no induced molting and beak trimming is decided on a case-by-case basis by the farmer; and (6) USDA certification.

Beyond Natural   The term "natural" doesn't mean much for eggs—according to the USDA, natural eggs are free of additives and colors. And according to the FDA, such practices are forbidden in shell eggs—so the term is contradictory and meaningless at best.

To satisfy their customers' interests, health-food stores have their own definition of "natural" and assigned staff or consultants, called standards experts, to make certain the claims are true. While this is not a perfect system, these self-described retail food police have a workable understanding of farming practices, and most health-food stores make sure that any eggs sold in their store meet the agreed-upon definition. They will not allow brands that use antibiotics or animal by-products in feed or allow cages and induced molting.

For the conventional grocery industry the descriptive labels attract consumers to higher-priced eggs; however, only a smattering of high-end specialty stores have systems in place to verify if the claims are true or have any credibility. Some of the health-food store brands are now in conventional grocery stores; read the fine print for words like "no antibiotics," "no cages," and "vegetarian-fed" and ignore the word "natural."

Biodynamic Farming   Biodynamic farming is a nongovernmental certified program for sustainable farming. This means the farmer must use approved farming methods that have the least environmental impact on the land possible. Biodynamic farmers adopt lifestyles that strive to preserve water, energy, and the surrounding natural habitat and observe farming methods that allow natural livestock. Specific to egg-laying hens: they must be outdoors as much as possible; vegetarian-fed (80% of feed must be produced on the farm); and subjected to no growth-promoting antibiotics or practices such as beak trimming and induced molting.

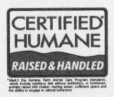

Certified Humane   This label is from an organization called Humane Farm Animal Care, which is supported by foundations such as the ASPCA and the HSUS. With the support of USDA certifiers, the group verifies that farms meet specific criteria for the humane treatment of hens. Practices include cage-free environments with natural living space, an environment that allows for natural behaviors like preening and scratching, vegetarian feed, and no antibiotics in feed. All eggs sold at Wild Oats grocers are Certified Humane.

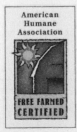

Free Farmed   Free-farmed-certified hens and their eggs provide a guarantee that claims such as "free-range," "cage-free," and "no subtherapeutic antibiotics" are genuine. Farmers are required to develop safe waste management systems and clean living conditions. This label is certified by the AHA.

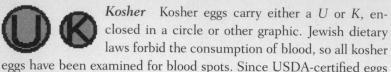

Kosher   Kosher eggs carry either a *U* or *K*, enclosed in a circle or other graphic. Jewish dietary laws forbid the consumption of blood, so all kosher eggs have been examined for blood spots. Since USDA-certified eggs are examined for this flaw, most government-certified brands are labeled as kosher. It is still common for Jewish cooks to check for bloodspots because once the blood-spotted egg hits the pan, the pan is no longer considered kosher.

OTHER ANIMAL WELFARE CLAIMS (NOT ALWAYS VERIFIED)

Cage-Free, Free-Roaming, or Free-Range   About 90% of American laying hens are raised in battery cages, wire cages that allow anywhere from forty-eight to sixty-eight square inches of space per hen, about the size of a sheet of computer paper. UEP says the confinement in battery cages protects the birds from harming one another and from the spread of diseases. UEP stands firm on its approval of wire cages for egg-laying hens.

Animal welfare experts disagree, saying that if only one change could be made to the U.S. egg industry it should be to ban battery cages, as they will be by 2012 in the E.U. The argument against them is that when hens no longer live in stressful conditions, salmonella rates and antibiotic needs decline.

According to the USDA and FDA, "cage-free" means the birds live outside cages but are still confined to an enclosed building. Some egg producers use the term "free-roaming" to mean the same thing as "cage-free."

We'd all like to believe that "free-range" means that hens spend the day basking in the sun, roaming in the grass, and clustering around Grandma's feet as she throws handfuls of Nebraska-grown corn from her apron pockets, but no such luck. The hens may have access to the outdoors, but they may actually never venture out the barn door. Most hens like to stay close to their nests, food, and water.

One of the arguments against free-range hens is that they are exposed to avian diseases from migratory fowl and salmonella from rodents, making free-range more inhumane than cages. "Inhumane" may be overstating it, but if bird flu continues to be a health problem, "cage-free" may become a more relevant term until the threat is gone. Since all of these terms, "free-roaming," "cage-free," and "free-range" are sometimes used interchangeably, undoubtedly this one label can be easily misinterpreted by consumers.

Grass-Fed, Grass-Ranged, or Pastured Hens   There is no USDA-approved term for 100% grass-fed egg-laying hens, nor will there be anytime soon. Unlike cows and sheep, which can live quite nicely on a diet of only grass, chickens cannot—they need protein. If left to their own devices they eat bugs for protein. Most often the hens are fed a ration of legumes, grains, fish meal, vitamins and minerals, and a bit of corn. So while you may see marketing terms such as "100% grass-fed egg-laying hens," it's not biologically possible, nor is it good for the hens.

A more accurate term is "pastured hens"; however, the conditions vary significantly. Egg layers need a coop for egg laying and protection from predators and the weather. This might be an open barn with coops for egg laying or small individual living spaces like enriched cages or small henhouses that are moved around to fresh patches of grassy land.

Most often eggs from pastured hens are sold at farmers' markets or small health-food stores, where consumers and store owners have direct access to the farmer. If you are genuinely concerned about the living conditions of egg-laying hens, ask the farmer questions about his or her farming methods. Since there are no agreed-upon definitions, the situations may vary. Better yet, if you really care about this, forgo the store and go directly to the farm; that way you can see first-hand how the hens are raised. Just make sure the eggs are clean and refrigerated.

Raised Without Antibiotics   The term "raised without antibiotics" is approved by the USDA, providing the farm shows paperwork proving the claim and removes any birds from the flock who are given antibiotics. This label is only as good as the frequency of the auditing. If this is important to you, ask your grocery store manager if he or she has a paperwork trail or system to verify whether the term "raised without antibiotics" is a true claim or not. This claim can legitimately be made for eggs that are certified as organic and biodynamic.

Vegetarian-Fed   If left to their own survival, chickens eat grains, grasses, and bugs for protein. On the farm, chickens are fed manmade feed that may contain animal or fish proteins along with grains or be solely vegetarian, eating a diet that includes grains, corn, cottonseed, and soybean meal.

In a roundabout way, the practice of feeding chickens animal protein could have reintroduced BSE back into the beef industry. It's a perfect example of the cyclical spread of an infectious agent. Here is how: protein for chicken feed may come from cattle by-products, which could be infected with BSE. When it's time to clean the barn, the litter (feathers, bedding, spilled feed, and feces) could have been sold back to the animal feed industry for cattle feed, which could in rare cases reintroduce BSE. This potential cycle of infections was broken in 2004 when the practice of using chicken litter to make cattle feed was banned.

READ THESE LABELS WITH A CRITICAL EYE

The following labels may indeed have merit or not. This is a gray area of egg labeling. It's important to know the integrity of an individual company or the level of oversight to determine whether the farming practices behind the statement are valid.

Antibiotic-Free   Although this term is used, "antibiotic-free" is not an approved USDA label, and rightly so, because it leaves a lot of room for interpretation. For some companies, "antibiotic-free" may mean that the hens have never been given antibiotics, ever. For others, the term can mean that the eggs were brought to market with less than traceable levels of antibiotics—not necessarily that the hens never received antibiotics. Remember, all hens treated with antibiotics must go through a withdrawal period before their eggs can be sold, which is why some processors would like to claim their eggs are antibiotic free.

Additive-Free, No Additives or Chemicals Added   For meat and poultry labels, the words "no additives or chemicals" mean that no ingredients have been added to the final product. In the case of eggs, additives such as colors are prohibited in egg production anyway and the hard shell prevents chemicals from being inserted into the eggs. These terms have nothing to do with whether pesticides or antibiotics were added to feed or administered to flocks.

Farm Fresh   All eggs are raised on farms of one size or another, with an assortment of farming practices—so it's not clear what this label implies.

Fertile Eggs   Fertile eggs are laid by hens that live in uncaged environments with roosters roaming about. These eggs are more perishable than unfertile eggs and therefore require special handling and may not last as long in the refrigerator. USDA and state egg inspectors throw fertile eggs away.

Fertile eggs may contain slightly higher levels of male hormones, but they are not significantly more nutritious than unfertile eggs, unless, say, the hens were grass-fed or given specialized feed to improve the fat profile—but this has more to do with feed than fertility. Fertile eggs are sold mostly by egg farms too small for the purview of state and federal inspectors (less than 3,000 hens). If anything, this label is a true indicator of an egg farm being cage-free, since the rooster has to be let in the henhouse to mingle.

Hormone-Free and Steroid-Free   In Colorado, I am fortunate to have staples like milk and eggs delivered to my doorstep weekly. One afternoon, a zealous salesman came by to convince me to switch to his delivery company. Just as I was about to politely decline and shut the door, he burst out with one more sales pitch: ". . . and our eggs are hormone-free."

Poor guy, he picked the wrong house to try that one. I tried not to shoot the messenger and explained that the use of hormones in poultry had been banned for more than forty years and that he would have to find a better, if not more legitimate, sales tactic.

Hormones are not allowed in any poultry-raising operations. If the label says "hormone-free" or "steroid-free," that should be followed with a disclaimer saying: "Federal regulations prohibit the use of hormones in poultry." However, this is not always visible or even present.

Natural   We can all agree that eggs are perhaps one of nature's most perfect natural protein sources, but when the term is applied to eggs, "natural" means nothing. The word "natural" is perhaps the most misleading label of all, because it implies that the hens were raised in a similar manner to organic hens, with no antibiotics or pesticides. By government standards the label means no artificial flavoring, colors, chemical preservatives, or artificial or synthetic ingredients have been added to the egg and it's minimally processed. But since FDA regulations prohibit additives or preservatives in eggs, this label means nothing. Unless they have been pasteurized or irradiated, all eggs are natural.

Bottom Line

Egg labels take a lot of time to digest and understand. More than any other food, the types of eggs you buy and the labels you pay attention to are a good indicator of the issues that you consider important, whether animal welfare, food safety, or health. Remember, though, that hormone-free eggs are a marketing ploy and "free-range" and "free-roaming" may not mean the same thing to all producers. And with the exception of pasteurized or irradiated eggs, all shell eggs are considered by the USDA to be natural and free of additives and colors.

One of the models for change in the egg industry came from an unlikely source, McDonald's, the world's largest egg buyer (more than 2 billion per year). The company told its suppliers to improve, or else. None waited for the "or else." In eighteen months, cage space was bumped up to seventy-two inches, beak cutting changed to trimming, and induced molting by starvation was banned (the guidelines were based on UEP's certification program). Even the animal rights groups who organized campaigns like chaining protesters to drive-up windows and painting Happy Meal toys a very unhappy bloody red were surprised by the improvements. Getting rid of the cages is still favored—but it's not likely to happen anytime soon. Even so, after decades of talking about what could and couldn't be done, in less than two years Mc-Donald's forced the issue. Not surprisingly, Burger King and Wendy's announced similar plans.

Most of the egg producers I spoke with said they wanted more federally approved guidelines for egg labeling, if for no other reason than to level the playing field and decrease consumer confusion. But sans federal monitoring or third-party verification for all egg farms, the industry is free to continue to use labels as a marketing net to catch consumers, who, as they reach for their weekly dozen, hope they are buying a safe and healthy food, contributing to the well-being of the hens, and supporting farmers who allow their hens to behave more like chickens and less like egg factory workers.

HEALTHY EGG LABELS

With designer eggs, labeled as having less cholesterol and less saturated fat and being high in omega-3, DHA (docosahexaenoic acid, a healthy fat found in fish), and vitamin E, it's hard to believe that eggs were at one time on the top of the cardiologist's list of food to avoid or eat sparingly. Updated research crossed them off the nutrition warning list, and improvements in agronomy opened the market to a new generation of designer eggs, with health benefits that parallel those of fish, known for essential fatty acids that improve heart health.

Eggs are loaded with a trio of healthy benefits: Choline helps with fetal brain development and decreases in memory loss later in life, and lutein and zeaxanthin are responsible for reducing free-radical damage in the eyes and preventing hardening of the arteries. Unless you are on a very restrictive diet, prescribed by your physician, eggs are recommended as part of a balanced diet.

Hens that lay the modern-day equivalent of the proverbial golden egg are fed a specialized diet of sea kelp, flaxseed, marigold petals,

(continued)

and healthy oils. Research shows that these nutritionally pampered hens lay eggs that are lower in cholesterol and saturated fat, as well as being higher in essential fatty acids such as omega-3, known to reduce sudden heart attack risk.

If you don't eat fish, eggs rich in DHA can be a good source of healthy omega-3 fatty acids. They cost almost double the price of other eggs but are still less expensive than fish. For instance, a dozen eggs with enhanced DHA cost about $3.99 and one serving of wild salmon (three ounces) can cost at least that much. Gram for gram the salmon contains 1 to 1.8g of omega-3 fatty acids, while two of the DHA designer eggs may contain up to 1.2g of omega-3s, depending on the brand.

Some egg brands use flaxseed in the chicken feed, which increases another type of omega-3 healthy fatty acid called alpha-linolenic acid (ALA). This is also a healthy fat; however, the body needs much more of it than DHA for a heart-healthy response.

BROWN EGGS

Eggshell color is not an indicator of health, quality, animal welfare, or taste—it's a preference. Eggshell color is determined by the breed of hens. White-shelled eggs are from white leghorn chickens (with white earlobes); brown eggs are from breeds like Rhode Island Reds (with brown earlobes); and blue eggs, found mostly in farmers' markets, are from South American Araucanas.

CHAPTER 5

Sea of Labels: Fish

Eat Fish, but Hold the Mercury, Please

"Since when is Atlantic salmon farmed fish?" my neighbor Lauren yelled over the back fence.

"Forever . . . at least for a long while," I yelled back, "You knew that, right?"

"No, but I do now. A lady scolded me in the seafood section for buying farmed salmon because of mercury. Right there in front of the mahimahi and the kids," she said.

I'm a little worried that our grocery store is becoming a soapbox for bad manners (I'm guilty as well). The reprimanding woman was probably trying to draw Lauren's attention to the FDA warnings about fish and mercury. Lauren was pregnant and pushing a two-year-old *and* a four-year-old in the grocery cart. She *is* the demographic the FDA targeted in their latest warnings about seafood.

Was the scolding warranted? First, the nosy shopper had it wrong—there are few troubles with salmon and mercury; salmon has a whole other set of problems related to heavy metals (polychlorinated biphenyls, more commonly known as PCBs). But for larger predatory fish (like swordfish), mercury is a problem.

If you've turned away from eating fish because the distinctions between risk and safety are too difficult to have down pat, please reconsider. A diet that includes fish plays an important role in good health. It's no secret that the Mediterranean diet is one of the healthiest—fish is one of the reasons for its fine standing reputation. Fish eaters show evidence of healthier triglyceride levels, reduced blood pressure, and a lowered risk of blood clots, stroke, and sudden death from heart attacks.

The caveat to all the good news is pollution, namely mercury, in our waterways and oceans, as well as countries halfway around the globe. Most of the mercury is attributed to airborne residues from coal-burning power plants, which travel through the jet stream and rain down into oceans, rivers, and lakes. Large fish with the highest stature on the food chain are most at risk for toxic levels of mercury for two reasons—they eat large quantities of other fish, and they live longer. All fish, though, contain some amount of mercury, so no fish is perfectly free from pollutants. It's a matter of degree.

The medical community has long warned that mercury is a proven human health risk that can cause neurological, cognitive damage and death, especially in infants and young children. Just how to warn American consumers that certain fish are carriers of mercury without decreasing our consumption of fish is a sticking point for the FDA, especially for canned tuna.

In 2001, the FDA issued a mercury warning that pregnant women should avoid swordfish, shark, king mackerel, and tilefish because of risk to the fetus for neurological damage. The FDA warning made the point that twelve ounces of *any other* fish per week was fine. The problem was, for many Americans *any other fish* means tuna, and it was absent from the list. Per capita, Americans eat almost nine six-ounce cans of tuna per year—that's nearly three tuna sandwiches a month or more tuna noodle casseroles than I care to calculate.

The omission raised concern that perhaps the FDA was buckling to pressure from the tuna industry. A report by the National Academy of Science insinuated that to protect the most vulnerable—pregnant women and children—*all* fish with unacceptable mercury levels should be on the list, no matter how popular. That meant albacore ("white") tuna should be on the warning list.

In February 2004, the EPA estimated that as many as 630,000 children are born each year with a risk for lowered intelligence and learning problems due to exposure to mercury. Although diet isn't the only source of exposure, a month later the FDA finally agreed to place albacore tuna on the warning list. Here is the recommendation from the FDA and EPA for women of childbearing age, pregnant women, and young children:

1. Do not eat shark, swordfish, king mackerel, or tilefish because they contain high levels of mercury.

2. Eat up to twelve ounces (two average meals) a week of a variety of fish and shellfish that are lower in mercury.

   - Five of the most commonly eaten fish that are low in mercury are shrimp, canned light tuna, salmon, pollock, and catfish.
   - Another commonly eaten fish, albacore tuna, has more mercury than canned light tuna. So when choosing your two meals of fish and shellfish, you may eat up to six ounces (one average meal) of albacore tuna per week.

3. Check local advisories about the safety of fish caught by family and friends in your local lakes, rivers, and coastal areas. If no advice is available, eat up to six ounces (one average meal) per week of fish you catch from local waters, but don't consume any other fish during that week.

If you eat tuna, read the preceding warning carefully and notice the bullet point in number 2: "Albacore tuna has more mercury than *canned light tuna.*" If you are pregnant, ever plan to get pregnant, or have young children who eat tuna, the FDA recommends that you stay within the six-ounce limit per week of albacore tuna.

However, Consumers Union says even these recommendations may be misleading. The group randomly tested light tuna for mercury and found that 6% exceeded the average mercury levels for albacore and some tested as high as .85 part per million (ppm), just a sliver below the FDA 1 ppm maximum safe limit. In this case, the mercury culprit is yellowfin tuna, which is sometimes packed with albacore tuna. Since the tests, the consumer group has suggested that pregnant women avoid eating canned tuna.

The FDA responded by noting that since mercury exposure is a cumulative problem, the occasional single serving that exceeded safety limits shouldn't be a problem. Again they noted that the cardiovascular benefits of eating fish outweigh the risk. Consumers Union disagrees, saying the uncertainty of whether brief exposure could cause harm is enough to warrant restraint during pregnancy. For children under forty-five pounds, Consumers Union recommends one-half to one six-ounce can of light tuna per week or up to one-third a can of albacore tuna per week (as long as no other mercury-containing seafood is eaten during that time). See the "Mercury in Fish" card reproduced in the shopping list appendix.

Is Wild Salmon Better, or Is That Just Another Fish Tale?

The argument about whether wild or farmed salmon is more contaminated with PCBs opens a big can of worms. It all comes down to PCBs, dioxins, and flame retardants. The toxins collect in the fat that permeates the meat and lies just under the salmon's skin. Some of the pollutants have been banned since the 1970s, but they still remain in the sediment; others leach out from waste dumps. Scientists are unsure how flame retardants, added to items like foam car seats and clothing for safety, get into salmon and other fish. Farmed salmon may contain even higher concentrations of contaminants because fish kibble (think of pet food for fish) is made from a concentration of millions of small fish.

Whether exposure to these contaminants over one's lifetime is high enough to warrant concern is not clear. Dioxins are known carcinogens; the risk for damage depends on how long one is exposed, at what age, and how often. Workers exposed to dioxins over long periods of time do show a higher rate of cancer. And dioxins are recognized by the National Academy of Science (NAC) as potentially damaging to the neurological systems of infants and babies in utero. It's disconcerting that nursing women in the United States have the highest dioxin levels in their breast milk in the world. Whether this adds up to health concerns is not well understood.

That said, improvements in emission reductions have reduced environmental exposure by more than 90% since 1987 by controlling major industrial sources including municipal and medical waste in-cinerators, hazardous waste incinerators, boilers and industrial fur-naces, and chlorine-bleaching pulp and paper mills.

Today the primary exposure source is our diet, because these chemi-cals break down very slowly in the environment. Even though emissions are down, dioxins remain in our groundwater and soil and concentrate in plants, the very same vegetation animals and fish eat. The chemicals concentrate in fats that we ingest—as much as 95% of our dioxin expo-sure comes from dietary fats. Although fish is one source of dioxins, it isn't the only source, as is seen in this NAC diagram.

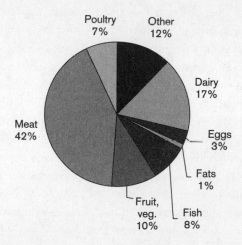

If meat and dairy are the top two dietary sources of dioxins, then why does farmed fish get the most negative press? The statistics point to beef as the number-one cause of exposure, because we eat more of it than fish. If we ate more fish than beef, the numbers could be eas-ily reversed. Also, the concentration of dioxins in farmed salmon is controllable through better feed formulations.

The farmed fish industry was the biggest target largely because of studies that show PCB and dioxin levels in farmed salmon from some regions exceed the cautionary limits for the EPA. A University of Albany study headed by Dr. David Carpenter tested more than two tons of salmon, wild and farmed, purchased at major cities in the

United States and Europe. The study pointed to farmed salmon as a health risk because PCB levels in fish from Scotland and the Faroe Islands exceeded the EPA's cautionary limits of 24 to 48 parts per billion (ppb), the highest reaching 36 ppb. U.S., Canadian, and Chilean salmon ranked significantly lower, depending on the source of the feed.

By EPA standards the test gave pause, but even our own government doesn't agree on what is worrisome. It's a matter of caught versus bought. The EPA oversees recreationally caught fish and the FDA monitors fish sold in grocery stores, setting the levels of concern as high as 2,000 ppb. The EPA bases their standards on the premise that if one eats only fish from streams and lakes known for high PCB levels, consumption should be limited. The FDA monitors the eating habits of grocery shoppers, not people who fish for their dinner. The assumption is that shoppers eat a variety of fish, from different sources, each with differing levels of contaminants.

The Albany study preferred the more conservative EPA numbers and went so far as to recommend that farmed salmon consumption be pared down to one serving or less per month for the highest contaminated sources. While physicians touted the health benefits of eating salmon, no matter the source, this was the first study that questioned the recommendation.

Not surprisingly, the farmed salmon industry jumped all over the study's validity. According to researchers from various backgrounds, there were flaws. The farmed salmon industry claimed that there were improvements in fish feed since the data was collected, which could have lowered the contaminant levels by one-third. And, when the fish was tested for toxins, researchers used a common method of grinding up the skin and the flesh. If the skin had been separated from the meat as most people do when eating fish, again, the contaminant levels would be lower.

Soon after the Albany study, Salmon of the Americas (SOTA), a farmed salmon association, presented its own study that compared Alaskan wild salmon with Canadian and U.S. farmed salmon. The PCB levels were virtually identical—8–11 ppb for both farmed and wild salmon.

The discrepancies between the Albany study and SOTA's sponsored study depend on where the salmon is raised and under what conditions. The Albany study was global in nature: Researchers tested salmon in the E.U., Canada, and the United States. American consumers have less to worry about than if one lives in Frankfurt, Edinburgh, Paris, or London—farmed salmon sold in these cities had the highest PCB and dioxin residues because it came from farms near Scotland and the Faroe Islands, where the fish consistently test higher for contaminants. Since most Americans eat farmed salmon from Chile and Canada, there should be much less concern than for Europeans.

But the controversy isn't over yet. To counter the negative press, SOTA came out with its own whopper of an advertising campaign. During the Thanksgiving week in 2005, SOTA ran a six-page advertorial in *The New York Times*. It featured a pregnant woman named Paula. Plastered across Paula's expanding belly was the slogan: "Ocean-Farmed Salmon . . . Just what the doctor ordered."

It's not surprising that the ad copy failed to note any suspicions about PCBs, flame retardants, or dioxins in farmed salmon. It's also not surprising that the National Environmental Trust, led by Dr. David Carpenter, author of the University of Albany study, filed an FTC complaint citing that the ad encouraged pregnant women to eat a food that places the brains of their developing fetuses at risk for irreversible damage. The FTC is reviewing the claims as this book goes to press.

So what should women like my neighbor do? At four dollars per pound, farmed salmon prices are tempting, especially if your doctor recommends eating fish for heart health and childhood development. Just like with the mercury warning for tuna, every cardiologist in this country is worried that the controversy will scare consumers away from eating fish. It hasn't happened for salmon; 22% of all grocery seafood sales are salmon (of any type). If you eat salmon and want to watch your intake of PCBs, here is what can be culled from experts:

1. If you chose not to eat fish at all because this is just too confusing, please reconsider. Your risk of developing heart disease by not eating fish is much higher than the possibility of developing cancer

from dioxins and PCBs in these fish. The threat of heart disease drops by one-third by putting fish on your menu twice a week. According to the EPA, if you ate farmed salmon once a month with PCB contaminant levels of up to 36 ppb for seventy years, your risk of getting cancer would be 1 out of 100,000.

2. Although the cancer risk is low, there are still no clear answers as to whether low-dose exposure to PCBs and dioxins will harm infants and young children. If you are pregnant and/or feeding small children and prefer to err on the side of caution, look for wild and farmed salmon that have been tested for contaminant levels (see the Seafood Watch certification program).

3. According to the most recent data released by the farmed salmon industry, PCB levels in farmed salmon from British Columbia, United States, and Chile average between 6.75 ppb to 11.5 ppb. Now that country-of-origin labeling is mandatory for seafood, there should be a sign in the seafood case telling you exactly where the fish came from. If it is missing, don't be embarrassed to ask— it's the law.

4. Given that wild salmon is relatively high on the fish food chain, this too has some degree of contamination, ranging from 5 ppb to 10 ppb. Since PCBs and dioxins collect in fat, lower-fat wild species may have the least contaminants (but also fewer heart-healthy fish oils). The fatty acid levels can change by the season and location, but in general wild salmon species in order of fatty acids from lowest to highest are chum, pink, Coho (silver), sockeye (red), and Chinook (King). Remember, the levels can vary significantly so there are no hard and fast rules.

   Wild salmon is seasonal; fresh sources are available only in the late spring through summer. If you are budget-minded, look for frozen wild salmon in the winter months; some brands are priced as competitively as farmed salmon. All canned salmon sold in the United States is wild.

5. In both categories of wild and farmed salmon, there are studies that show higher-than-average contamination rates from very spe-

cific regions, such as Copper River sockeye, Chinook from Washington's Puget Sound, and the farmed salmon from Faroe Islands. If you see reports that say wild salmon is significantly higher in contaminants than farmed, it is usually regarding sockeye and Chinook specifically from these areas. Chinook's size, which can exceed 100 pounds in weight, makes this species more susceptible to toxic residues. In addition, polluted sediments in lakes, rivers, and sounds can affect PCB and dioxin levels in some wild salmon.

If you see reports that say farmed salmon is significantly higher in contaminants, most likely it came from Scotland and Faroe Islands. Each side of the salmon industry likes to play these facts against the other. The bottom line is that if one looks in the right places for PCBs and dioxins, they are not hard to find.

6. Whether wild or farmed, remove the skin and the thin layer of fat beneath where the pollutants concentrate. This will reduce but not eliminate all the contaminants, since fats permeate throughout the flesh (toxins tend to accumulate in the fat).

7. Eat a variety of fish rather than salmon again and again. Other seafood with high levels of omega-3s (per three-ounce serving) include herring (1.7g), Atlantic mackerel (1g), farmed rainbow trout (.8–1g), sardines (.8g), swordfish and albacore tuna (.7–.9g, mind the mercury), halibut and mussels (.7g), crab, sole, and pollack (.4g). Shrimp, light tuna, catfish, clams, cod, and mahimahi contain .2g or less. See the *Eating Between the Lines* Shopping List at the back of this book for a mercury seafood chart.

Better Fish Farming and Sustainable Seas

From a health perspective, the issue of farmed versus wild isn't as clear-cut as fish lovers would like to believe. From an environmental perspective, the issues aren't any simpler. Salmon farming's reputation—that it isn't the kindest, most gentle system on the environment—was well-documented in the 1980s and 1990s. It took three to five pounds of small fish to make a pound of salmon, which can take its toll on smaller-fish populations. Antibiotics were not prohibited or used with restraint. And there were concerns that waste from these liquid farms polluted the surrounding aqua systems. Escaping fish was also a concern.

Even though there is still resistance to the farmed salmon industry, the situation today has improved. It is not a perfect system, and there are still mindsets among some consumers and environmentalists against farmed salmon. However, according to new statistics released in Canada by the farmed salmon industry (few were available for U.S. fisheries), in this new era of fish farming it takes about 1.14 tons of fish to produce 1 ton of farmed salmon because of improvements in feed formulations; antibiotic use is down to .3mg per two pounds of fish (withdrawal periods are mandatory); and about 2.5% of feed is premedicated. Fish escapes in North America have dropped dramatically from hundreds of thousands per year to isolated cases because of improvements in net technology.

A continuing problem is algal blooms, when some algae species multiply so quickly that the caged fish are cut off from oxygen. Wild fish are less affected because they can escape the affected area. In the last five years, hundreds of thousands of pounds of farmed fish and shellfish have been killed by the rapidly growing slimy green algae. In addition to killing fish, certain algae species may also be incapacitating and killing marine mammals, particularly the California sea lions, whales, and dolphins. When these animals eat fish that consume algae, like anchovies and sardines, the mammals are poisoned by a neurotoxin that damages the animals' brain function.

NASA has been collecting satellite images of the massive blooms, which have spread from Chile in the southern hemisphere to as far north as Norway and throughout the Pacific Ocean. Critics of aquaculture blamed the increased levels on fish farms, but a single cause is not apparent. Large-scale blooms off the coast of England were reported in regions where there is no fish farming. Blooms near Florida's coast are believed to be triggered by dust storms from the Sahara desert. Japanese researchers attribute theirs to lightning strikes, which can alter nitrogen levels in seawater to create ideal conditions. The Scottish government is exploring multiple causes, including whether the flora remain hidden until the conditions are just so. The triggers may be changes in water temperature, increased nitrogen from land-based farm run-off, as well as human errors in fish farming.

Given the issues of finding clean and abundant feed, disease risk, and rampant algae blooms, is it possible to raise salmon even more sustainably than this? Absolutely, it just costs more than the low prices we've become accustomed to. It costs more to avoid antibiotics entirely because net square footage needs to be smaller. And it costs more to develop new feed formulations with fewer toxins and less dependency on small-fish populations. It also costs more to create impenetrable habitats that prevent fish from escaping.

Where some see obstacles, others see opportunity. One company that is trying to rise above the fray between environmental activists and farmed salmon's ill-fated reputation is Creative Salmon in Clayoquot Sound, British Columbia. In 2000, the company took a chance and did the unthinkable: They stopped using antibiotics on a portion of their stock. "We were told right away by veterinarians and feed salesmen that it was too risky," says Neil MacLeod, director of business development. The fish survived quite nicely. It was an issue of density. "Once the fish were less stressed, there was virtually no disease."

As of October 2001, the company stopped using antibiotics altogether, as well other pollutants like copper-dipped nets that can destroy life on the sea floor, and harsh drugs to treat sea lice. In the end, Creative Salmon proved the doubters wrong, and the fish got bigger, which has proved to be an economic payoff for the small forty-five-person company, MacLeod says. Creative Salmon used this knowledge to begin the process of developing organic standards for farmed salmon in Canada.

Even with company efforts to raise salmon sustainably there are some who prefer that the fishery operate in closed tanks rather than in open water. Creative Salmon's home port, Tofini, in Clayoquot Sound, is an environmental preservation site that is revered by First Nations' Indians, the region's native inhabitants. The two groups work in relative harmony with each other. The area is also home to an environmental group, Friends of the Clayoquot Sound, which is against open-sea salmon farming, no matter how sustainable. The organization wants salmon farming restricted to closed-tank systems, which is the newest evolution in fish farming. This may be an option for some fisheries, but Creative Salmon believes it is possible to raise salmon in open waters while still respecting the environment.

MacLeod says the biggest lesson the company has learned is thanks to operating in an environment that is a public resort and a preservation site, that transparency and respect are paramount. During the mid-1980s, when farmed salmon was a new industry, this philosophy was absent from many operations. Instead, MacLeod says, it was a "gold-rush mentality," which is how the industry got its "black eye" for careless use of antibiotics, escaping fish, and contaminated feed.

Also in the early years, fish farming wasn't a structured industry, per se; it was a hodgepodge of hundreds of small operations with no capital to invest in equipment or the know-how to predict the environmental impact of escaping fish, waste products, and contaminated feed. If one can make a first impression only once, this was the era that created the most adversity.

Today, there are only six companies that dominate the farmed-salmon industry. The corporate offices are in Norway, Chile, Holland, and Scotland, an ocean away from North American waters. The mere size and political power of these corporations adds to the tension between activist groups and the farmed-salmon industry.

Whether one is a supporter of corporate fish farming or not, the capital investments within North American operations transformed the industry. Million-dollar cages with impenetrable layers, which can stand up to predators and the torments of the sea, replaced the homemade flimsy counterparts. Scientifically developed feed, made up of a combination of fish by-products, grains, and small fish, is now the norm, rather than concentrated kibble with high toxin levels. This is not to say there aren't still valid concerns. Diseases, water effluence, waste, and good old human error are still obstacles and serious environmental challenges in the fish-farming industry.

In this author's opinion, perhaps the biggest disappointment is that during its inception years this new trade failed to learn from the history and mistakes of other farming industries. Here was an entirely new food system, with entirely new possibilities, using the same old philosophy of cheap and easy. Industry pioneers could have gained market share and consumer confidence by looking at poultry production and the real cost of antibiotic abuse, cattle ranching and feed science, or egg farming and the hazards of confinement. Instead, salmon aquaculture farms are backtracking to try to clean up their tainted reputations.

In addition, salmon fisheries using cleaner practices, like Creative Salmon, find it difficult to overcome the disastrous decisions of the past. MacLeod says that it costs at least 50% more in production costs to raise farmed salmon sustainably. The challenge is that consumers have either become accustomed to such low prices with conventionally raised salmon they can't justify the higher prices, or they have turned away from farmed salmon completely because they are bewildered by the complexity of the issue. If asked, "Is wild or farmed salmon better?" there isn't one single answer.

There are some who continue to argue that open-water fish farming should never be allowed. But it's doubtful that fish farming will go away and, in truth, it is necessary. The oceans can't bear the burden of consumer demand for all types of seafood. Fish farming is necessary; it just doesn't have to be a necessary evil. This country's reliance on seafood imports and the resultant trade deficit is second only to oil. Nearly 70% of the seafood consumed in this country is imported and of this, 40% is farmed. China dominates most of the aquaculture market—44.3 million tons, as compared to the second highest, Peru, at 8.5 million tons. The concern from food- and marine-safety experts is, the Chinese fishing industry lacks the safety standards U.S. consumers expect. The only way to overcome this is to establish our own sizable U.S. aquaculture system, with our own conservation rules to better support eco-minded operations.

In the summer of 2006, legislation was proposed to begin offshore aquaculture in the United States. There are fears that this will once again create a Wild West mentality, which is why many are calling for approval of specific statutes to address how this will impact the seas before permits and leases are approved. California lawmakers are trying to stay one step ahead of another gold-rush situation. In summer of

2006, the California legislature passed formal aquaculture controls, which will minimize the use of chemical pesticides, create guidelines for fishmeal composition, and mandate careful oversight to prevent the spread of disease and penned fish from escaping into the wild.

I recently saw a supermarket ad that summed up how ludicrous these issues have become for consumers. The Wednesday shopper flyer said WILD SWORDFISH. I flinched when I read it—"wild" seemed ridiculous and redundant in the same sentence with "swordfish." Who would have imagined that one of the wildest fish known to man and sea would be marketed as wild, as if there was another type of swordfish?

Above all, when you are shopping for fish, keep in mind that not all fish can be, or should be, farmed, and that not all fishing operations are damaging to the environment. In this country, there are examples of rainbow trout, mollusk, shrimp, and tilapia farming that have proven their merit both environmentally and economically. Now the challenge is to apply the best practices across the industry.

One illustration as a positive force for change is the Open Ocean Aquaculture Demonstration Project experiment in the deep sea off the coast of New Hampshire (a National Oceanic & Atmospheric Administration [NOAA] project). It's a modern-day Jonny Quest and Jacques Cousteau in one. This undersea fish-farming video game uses a remote control measuring system, which tells the researchers exactly when the fish are hungry, their preferred water temperatures, and about other sea world comforts. The first experiments raised a ton and a half of cod in a region that had been void of commercial fishing for more than fifty years, with no negative environmental impact. The technology is still too expensive for commercial use, but think of where we might be today had the fish-farming industry started here in the first place. See the Addendum in the back for an update.

Seafood Labels

SEAFOOD LISTS

Have you ever stood at the fish counter in your supermarket fishing through your wallet, looking for that card that tells you the most environmentally conscious choices in the seafood case? What you may not have noticed was the grocery clerk behind the counter with drops of sweat collecting across his brow and along the brim of his supermarket-issued cap, nervously waiting for the grilling.

The most popular list is the Monterey Bay Aquarium's Seafood Watch. I have nothing against such lists or the groups that create them. The Monterey Bay Aquarium is a veritable Disneyland of marine life and the staff works hard to be protectors of ocean life. The Seafood Watch lists are well researched and can direct consumers toward choices that don't negatively impact already fragile marine ecosystems. However, other lists are not updated as frequently as the Seafood Watch list, nor are they as specific as they should be (for the most current Seafood Watch list, go to www.mbayaq.org).

Despite good intentions, these lists can make fish clerks in the supermarket very nervous. Unless you are in a more progressive grocery store, where the fishmongers practically have Ph.D.s in the subject, this clerk may have worked in the produce section only since last week. He knows that card may incite finger-pointing and questions like "Is that caught with a pole or trawl?" and "Is that a wild Patagonian sea bass from Antarctica or a farmed striped sea bass from the Gulf of Mexico? . . . Now where is that card?"

It's doubtful that even we understand what all this really means. Why then, out of the blue, is this poor guy making ten dollars an hour (if he has a good union) expected to have the educational pedigree of a marine biologist and the pinpoint accuracy of an oceanographer's GPS system? Many of these finned, clawed, or bivalve creatures are on avoid lists for very complicated reasons, including overfishing (although not everyone agrees what even this is); the impact on by-catch (unintended catch of endangered species or fish with no commercial value); disagreements about the way the fish are caught (farmed versus wild or bottom dredged versus line caught) and where they are from—the Pacific or the Atlantic.

If you approach the fish counter with the expectation that every item on ice needs to be marshaled because it is endangered, relax. There are actually a lot of people who make sure many fish species are never caught, much less make it to the store. For instance, here are a few species that are on some avoid lists: swordfish, sturgeon, shark, halibut, and Chilean seabass. Don't bother trying to remember them all. Undersized swordfish is banned from being imported into this country; domestic sturgeon, many species of shark, and Atlantic halibut are on either the endangered-species list or species-of-concern list with NOAA. Chilean seabass has very strict import rules that are monitored by NOAA, as well. Other species may be listed in the avoid column because they are under the threat of being overfished, or because the way in which they are caught places other sea life, birds, or marine mammals at risk. This last category, approaching overfishing and by-catch, is perhaps the most useful purpose for these watch lists because at times our big government machine operates too slowly to force immediate modifications.

To better understand how certain species end up on these lists, it is essential to know the basics of U.S. fishery management. The Magnuson-Steven Act, which has been in place for thirty years, requires the identification of all habitats that are essential to spawning, breeding, feeding, and maturing of primary fish species. As of this writing the act is up for renewal; most parties involved are predicting reauthorization and calling it the strictest conservation law to date. Critics say new revisions allow for too much time to rebuild fish stocks.

The act mandates that NOAA map out all of home turf for coastal fish (sardines, mackerel, anchovy, jack mackerel, market squid), salmon, groundfish (rockfish, sablefish, flatfish, Pacific whiting), and migratory species (tuna, swordfish, and sharks). The management of these habitats is a collective effort between NOAA, eight regional Fishery Management Councils, private fishing companies, and federal and state agencies.

Once the habitats are accounted for, U.S. fishing operations are placed on a quota system. Individual Fishing Quotas (IFQs) are federal permits issued to individual fishing operations, allowing the company to harvest a quantifiable amount of fish. These quotas are highly controversial. On the positive side, IFQs reduce the problem of too many fishing boats and too much gear (called overcapitalization) and afford economic certainty for fishermen because they regulate the supply and demand.

On the downside, IFQs means not as many fishing boats, so some operations have closed up shop. IFQs must also be monitored carefully because the system creates a race mentality—who can catch the most fish first. Permits are based on historical catch rates—the bigger the operation, the larger the quota—which can lead to monopolies. And, if improperly monitored, unethical fishermen can abuse the system by underreporting by-catch (unintended catch) or throwing low-priced fish aside in favor of higher-priced fish (a practice called "highgrading").

No doubt you've heard it before, our hunger for fish is outpacing supply, which is leading to shortages and the decimation of certain species. In truth, the problem is less critical among U.S.-managed fisheries than foreign seas. According to the most recent FAO report in 2004, "The State of World Fisheries and Aquaculture," here is the current state of the global seas:

- 24% of the world's fish stocks are either underexploited (3%) or moderately exploited (21%); both terms mean they could supply more.
- 52% are fully exploited, meaning they are close to or at capacity.
- 16% are overexploited, 7% depleted, and 1% are recovering from depletion (24% total).

Of the top ten species that account for 30% of the world's capture fisheries production, seven are in this third category of overexploited, depleted, or recovering. The percentage of stocks that are exploited beyond their sustainable levels varies greatly by area. The regions with the most exploited stocks (fully or overexploited) are the western Indian Ocean (75% fully exploited) and Western Central (73% fully exploited) and Northeast (59%) Atlantic. The FAO says that overall, a global capacity of 80% has been reached. One of the primary causes of overfishing, the report says, is by-catch rates, which are extremely high in some regions because of a lack of selective fishery management and sufficient monitoring.

The terminology for U.S.-managed fish stocks is slightly different than that of the U.N. NOAA defines the status of marine fish stocks based on two variables, the harvest rates and the stock size. NOAA uses the following terms to track fish stocks:

Overfishing: The harvest rate is above a prescribed mortality threshold.
Overfished: The stock size is below a prescribed biomass threshold.
Approaching overfished: The fishery will become overfished within two years.

A species can be labeled with one or all of the criteria, depending on allowable harvest rates (IFQs) and how well known the optimum stock size is. Here are the latest 2005 figures for U.S.-managed fisheries:

- Overfishing: 81% of the known fish stocks are not subject to overfishing; 19% are experiencing overfishing, meaning the current harvest rate exceeds the threshold stock size.
- Overfished: 74% are not overfished (of these 4% were approaching overfished status) and 26% are overfished, meaning the stock size is not what it should be.

Overall these numbers are similar to the previous year's; some stocks improved while others declined. In a nutshell, about one quarter of the U.S. fish stocks are not of adequate size. If one digs down further into the data and looks at which types of fish are depleted, the primary concerns are cod and groundfish species such as snapper and grouper. The remaining stocks that are not overfished are fairly robust in quantity.

The intent here is not to confuse the issue or downplay the importance of maintaining marine fish stocks, but to clarify the magnitude of the problem. Globally, the problem is difficult to manage because each country has its own system, or lack thereof, of fishery management. Many of the disagreements in this country are a clash of two ideals—some marine conservationists would prefer a complete moratorium on 26% of the U.S. stocks that are experiencing overfishing. At the very least they want quicker action. Government officials say this "blue-zoo" philosophy isn't necessary for most species. They believe a

well-structured quota system is sufficient to allow for commercial via-
bility and steady progress toward restoration. The timeframe to restore overfished species can be anywhere from ten to forty-plus years,
which is a long time by most marine conservationist calendars.

A recent scrap among fishermen, conservationists, and government officials in Florida illustrates the difficulty. In June 2006,
NOAA proposed restricting the quotas for snapper, grouper, tilefish,
and black seabass for the South Atlantic region. Shrimp trawling had
taken its toll on the groundfish habitat; each year as many as 4 million
pounds of red snapper are killed by the weight of shrimp nets and
from entanglement.

Marine conservationists say the problem has been building for nine
long years, with no action. NOAA agreed, saying the issue needed to
be addressed, but the local Gulf Fishery Council, which is ultimately
responsible for the region, voted to delay any action because the region
had been hit hard by the ravages of Hurricane Katrina. Apparently, in
the marine world, "dire" and "salvageable" have different meanings depending on what side of the beach one works from.

Now back to the fish-buying lists. Unfortunately, there isn't enough
editorial space here to fully explain the arguments for each species, but
please don't assume that every fillet under glass and on ice should be
suspect or the retailer should be on a conservationists's "most wanted
list," especially if the fish is from U.S. fisheries. And there is never
enough space on the little watch card to point out specific sustainable
fisheries for both wild and farmed fish. Bear in mind that even though
certain species are on watch lists, there are companies that go to great
hardship and expense to find eco-friendly ways to bring all types of
seafood to market—companies like these deserve our support, not our
suspicion.

Also remember that federal monitoring prevents most endangered
and fraudulently labeled fish, especially imported seafood, from making it to your seafood counter. For example, in August 2006, two companies and an individual pleaded guilty to the mislabeling of more
than one million pounds of Vietnamese catfish. To avoid U.S. import
duties, the fish was falsely labeled as grouper, channa, snakehead,
and bass.

If you are passionate about such issues, stay informed—the livelihood of this country's fishing industry depends on it. Federally mandated quotas are as fluid as the sea; they change so frequently that outdated consumer messages and mindsets can harm business. For instance, do you remember the very popular "Give Swordfish a Break" campaign, in which restaurants and retailers refused to serve or sell the fish? This crusade sticks in consumers' minds, which, to be honest, is the definition of a perfectly executed public relations campaign.

The problem is, there is no campaign on the other side of success. For instance, within two years of the swordfish boycott movement, U.S. swordfish stores greatly improved. Domestic Atlantic supplies are now in quantities large enough to support the U.S. marketplace. Aside from the mercury warning, do you still avoid buying swordfish for fear of reprisal from a meddlesome shopper standing guard at the fish counter?

ECO-LABELS

The following labels are very useful when making a quick decision at the seafood counter, frozen case, or even canned section. The caveat (there seem to be a lot of them with seafood) is that some very conservation-minded companies may choose not to pay to participate in these labeling programs—but they may be as equally conscientious.

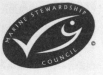 *The Marine Stewardship Council (MSC)* This was the first seafood eco-label, introduced in the 1990s. The program allows any size fishery to apply for the certification and uses independent certifiers to monitor compliance. Certifiers screen fisheries for the condition of the available stocks and the fisheries' impacts on the environment and management systems. MSC certification lasts for five years, with yearly audits. Certified products can be traced back directly to their source. You can find MSC-certified fresh, frozen, chilled, canned, and smoked seafood in grocery stores such as Safeway, Whole Foods, Wild Oats, and Wal-Mart.

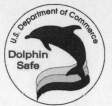 *The Dolphin-Safe Tuna* This label was perhaps the first of all eco-friendly labels to gain consumer compassion and interest. A generation that grew up with *Flipper* reruns after school strongly supported fishing standards that protected dolphins from demise. In 1991, the National Marine Fisheries Service (NMFS) implemented the dolphin-safe labeling system that protected dolphins from death during tuna fishing.

All was well until on New Year's Eve of 2002 the U.S. Department of Commerce tried to weaken the existing law by allowing tuna caught off the coast of Mexico to be imported to the United States. Current laws prohibit a common international fishing practice that chases down a school of dolphins, taking advantage of their precarious friendship with tuna, and encircles them in catch nets. The practice invariably ensnares dolphins as well.

In an unusual move, U.S. District Court judge Thelton E. Henderson agreed in August 2003 to roll back the laws to the original standards of the coveted Dolphin Safe label. The case, presented by the HSUS, the Earth Island Institute, and other conservation groups, proved to Henderson that the government was ignoring even their own studies that showed the dolphins were indeed endangered by these fishing methods. By Henderson's account, it was a clear case of buckling to political pressure.

The administration agreed to abide by the court decision as the final ruling. Tuna companies StarKist, Bumble Bee, and Chicken of the Sea stated that they would abide by the stricter "Dolphin Safe" standards indefinitely, despite any political countering. If by chance the laws are weakened again, the HSUS says they will immediately adopt a new label that is truly dolphin friendly.

By-Catch Program In 1989, a label called Turtle-Safe Certified was adopted to raise awareness about a problem called by-catch. The label highlighted shrimping operations that used netting called TEDS, which do not snare turtles. Unfortunately, the label is discontinued, but the issue is still relevant. The Sea Turtle Restoration Project

(STRP), founders of the label, were hopeful that U.S. laws requiring the nets and a ban on shrimp imports from nations that failed to adopt a TEDS shrimp-harvesting program would be enough to keep the turtles safe. The STRP says that due to difficulty in enforcement, shrimpers get around the law and do indeed catch sea turtles as by-catch.

The NOAA reports that for domestic operations TEDS exclude up to 97% of the sea turtles that could otherwise be caught in shrimp nets. Proving this high rate of success for international shrimp boats is more difficult. Each year the U.S. State Department recognizes countries that offer such safeguards and countries that do not comply are dropped from the list. However, STRP conservationists claim that the TEDS nets are sewn on for the inspections, which are preannounced, and removed when officials move on.

In March 2005 the U.S. Coast Guard and officials from the NOAA seized a Mexican fishing boat for such an act. The captain was sent to prison for sixteen months. In January 2006, NOAA law enforcement reported a similar incident with a U.S. shrimp boat. The STRP says these are just two of many examples of skirting the law.

By-catch is a looming problem in the fishing industry. For instance, scallop farming in the Mid-Atlantic snares too many sea turtles (749 in 2004), though new trawl nets introduced in summer 2006 will hopefully reduce this number. As mentioned earlier, trawl fishing that drags the sea bottom in the Gulf of Mexico also collects unwanted red snapper, rockfish, halibut, and skate, which can seriously deplete stores. To date, the most successful program to reduce by-catch is in the North Pacific Council, which oversees fisheries in the Bearing Sea, Aleutian Islands, and Gulf of Alaska. The Council requires procedures such as at-sea observers to track by-catch rates, fishing gear restrictions, fishery closures, and careful monitoring. The Marine Fish Conservation Network is calling for similar programs in all U.S. fishery councils, especially in the southern United States.

Buy U.S. Wild Shrimp   This isn't an official labeling program, but by purchasing wild shrimp collected from U.S. waters you can make a big difference for shrimpers. The Gulf Coast shrimping industry used to account for 10,000 boats and hundreds of other related packing and shipping businesses. That number has dwindled to a couple thousand boats. Hundreds of thousands of pounds of shrimp lie in the waters along the Gulf; however, Hurricane Katrina destroyed, much of the shrimping infrastructure. Competition waits for no one; fisheries have stepped in to meet the demand and now as much as 90% of the shrimp is imported from Asia. A campaign of U.S. shrimpers dubbed the Voyage of Food Independence is trying to nick away at this percentage (order shrimp directly from Gulf shrimpers, at www.american fishermansmarketing.com). The only caveat to this program is the problem of by-catch from Gulf shrimpers (as mentioned previously), but until the fishery management councils in the area decide to take positive action, this will be an ever-present problem and obstacle to attracting eco-minded consumers.

 Best Aquaculture Practices Certified   This certification system, which is overseen by the Aquaculture Certification Alliance, is an all-encompassing program that certifies domestic and imported shrimp farms and the processing plants. The seal not only means the shrimp were raised without antibiotics, in compliance with local environmental regulations, and in accordance with local and national labor laws; the label also means that the cleaning, packaging, and transporting practices are certified to meet Best Aquaculture Practices (BAP). The system offers complete traceability from the hatchery pond to the seafood case through Radio Frequency Identification (RFID), which is a computer chip placed in each tray of shrimp (you might call it the ultimate fish and chip—sorry, too good, or bad, to resist). As of this writing, BAP-certified shrimp are sold in Wal-Mart grocery stores and Whole Foods grocers (also served in Red Lobster, Olive Garden, and Bahama Breeze restaurants).

HEALTH AND FOOD SAFETY LABELS
With all the controversy surrounding fish, physicians fear that consumers will stop eating fish. So far that hasn't happened, which is a

good thing. If one is well aware of the types of fish that can be consumed safely, the risk from environmental pollutants is minimal.

Fish contain generous amounts of calcium, phosphorus, iodine, iron, and vitamins A and D. But their prime nutritional paybacks are two long-chain omega-3 fatty acids, called eicosapentaenoic acid (EPA) and DHA. Both of these fatty acids play a major role in heart and joint health, in addition to helping the body fight off cancers, reduce depression, and lower inflammation.

Health Claim: *Supportive but not conclusive research shows that consumption of EPA and DHA omega-3 fatty acids may reduce the risk of coronary heart disease.*

In 2004, the FDA approved this health claim for fish and dietary supplements, noting the importance of the two essential fatty acids, EPA and DHA, for heart health. The FDA recommends that consumers limit their consumption of omega-3 fatty acids to 3g per day from fish and 2g from fish oil supplements because both act as blood thinners.

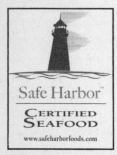

Safe Harbor   This newly developed label certifies that the seafood has been tested for mercury and the levels are among the lowest for each species. The label is a result of a new technology that measures mercury levels quickly and accurately. The company also offers an online calculator to measure your daily mercury exposure.

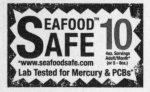

Seafood Safe   Seafood Safe labels are on all EcoFish-branded products. The label indicates how many four-ounce portions consumers can eat each month without ingesting potentially harmful levels of contaminants. For instance, a number 10 means one can consume 10 four-ounce servings per month. The labeling standard uses the EPA's guidelines, which are more stringent than those of the FDA and are set at a level that protects the most vulnerable adults—women of childbearing age. The products are randomly tested through independent laboratories for mercury and PCB levels.

Organic Seafood   Despite what you may see on food packaging and restaurant menus, there is no federal USDA organic-certified seafood. Even so, there is nothing to prevent a company from selling their product as organic—as long as the official USDA organic seal is not used. Some states, such as Florida, have their own USDA organic seafood certification process, which is why you may see, for instance, frozen organic shrimp. Moreover, some foreign countries have organic seafood certification and sell their fish in this country as organic.

There is resistance to this practice since uniformity is lacking and consumers now expect a certain assurance from even the word "organic." California law recently banned the sale of any organically labeled seafood until state or federal standards are endorsed. The National Organic Standards Board (NOSB) has begun the review process for organic seafood certification. The domestic "organic" shrimp-farming industry is pushing for a USDA organic-certified label because international conventional shrimp farms can be known for liberal use of antibiotics. It is not known whether certified organic seafood will have to comply with a minimum level of contaminants, such as mercury or PCBs.

OTHER FISH FACT LABELS

Color added refers to a practice of putting color additives in fish feed. Canthaxanthin and astaxanthin, from beta-carotene, give the fish an orange color. Canthaxanthin is also used in chicken feed, to color the chicken flesh yellow.

Previously frozen fish must be labeled accordingly. Previously frozen fish cannot be refrozen unless it is first cooked.

Flash frozen utilizes a quick freezing method that takes place on fishing trawlers, allowing the seafood to be frozen within two hours of catch and in as little as three seconds. The seafood is packed and shipped frozen, held in subzero freezers, and never thawed.

The country of origin label (COOL) is now mandatory for fresh and frozen seafood. The ruling requires seafood to be labeled wild, instead of ocean caught, and that the word "farmed" be added to the "Atlantic" salmon label. The labeling change means more paperwork and record keeping; however, the extra work can help identify fish that needs to be recalled. For instance, only a few months after the COOL labeling, the FDA recalled Vietnamese *basa* catfish sold in Alabama, Mississippi, Louisiana, and Florida because of an antibiotic not approved for use in aquaculture.

Bottom Line

There is an African proverb that says filthy water cannot be washed. Perhaps the greatest paradox in trying to feed humans from the sea is that the consequences of our actions on land are inescapably tied to the oceans. The very water that feeds us can also poison us.

Regardless of whether we rely on traditional fishermen or farmed fisheries for our food, irresponsible actions are intolerable. Equally intolerable are out-of-reach expectations that cannot be met. Fish farming does manipulate the environment, as do all types of farming, but not all fish farming is appalling, as consumers are sometimes led to believe. The fish-farming industry has a responsibility to apply the most stringent standards possible; low cost is not an excuse for bad business practices.

It's equally vital to understand that not all wild fish are on the brink of extinction, especially among U.S.-managed fisheries. There are exceptions that must be dealt with accordingly, but fear mongering is a poor way to gain attention and public support for a cause as important as the health of our seas and its inhabitants.

Paul Hawkin says, in his book, *The Ecology of Commerce*: "Just as every act in an industrial society leads to environmental degradation, regardless of intention, we must design a system where the opposite is true, where doing good is like falling off a log, where the natural, everyday acts of work and life accumulate into a better world as a matter of course, not a matter of conscious altruism." In this author's opinion, there is no better place to start than with the sea and a food as important to our health as seafood.

TIPS FOR FISHING AT THE SUPERMARKET

1. **Look for Freshness:** Ask the seafood manager which day of the week seafood is delivered to the store and buy on those days. Fresh fish fillets should have a moist, bright surface; old fish is dry and dull. Whole fish should have clear eyes, bright pink gills, and shiny, attached scales. Fish should smell like the sea, not fishy. If even fresh, unspoiled fish still smells unappealing to you, soak it in a milk bath with a few lemon slices for ten minutes.

2. **Ask Questions:** If you don't see what you want, ask for it. Usually the seafood department has an extensive catalog of choices that can be ordered. Be sure to check on the price, though, as out-of-season fish can be extraordinarily expensive.

3. **Check the Dates:** Don't buy seafood past the expiration date. Prepackaged seafood has a sell-by or use-before date. A sell-by date indicates how long the product should remain on the shelves. A use-before date is the last date you should consume the product.

4. **Cook or Freeze:** It's best to cook fish on the day of purchase. It can be chilled for two days at the most. Freeze for up to six months. Defrost frozen seafood in the refrigerator just before cooking. Cook frozen fish within a day of defrosting.

5. **Avoid Contamination:** Use different cutting boards and separate knives when preparing raw fish. Wash your hands often, as well as all of the utensils and contact surfaces.

6. **Don't Overcook:** Allow ten minutes of cooking time for every inch of thickness for medium-cooked fish. The flesh should flake easily when done and be opaque throughout. Salmon and tuna can be cooked to medium rare. Cook all other fish to 145 degrees Fahrenheit.

SUPERMARKET SUSHI

My first taste of sashimi was at 5:00 A.M. at the Tsukiji fish market in Tokyo. With the precision of a surgeon, a vendor carved off a coral-colored sliver of tuna for me to try. With a polite bow, I accepted. My twenty-year-old brain could barely comprehend the experience—the taste was primal, sweet, and clean. For the rest of the morning I sipped hot green tea in a nearby fishermen's sushi bar and ate whatever sweet morsels from the sea were artfully placed before me.

Since that day, I've naturally been leery about eating raw fish at inland restaurants, much less at grocery stores, and certainly not out of the grab-and-go case at a convenience store. Is my skepticism warranted? First let's clarify some terms. Sushi is not raw fish. "Sushi" means vinegary rice that is rolled with vegetables, fish, or pickled vegetables, wrapped in seaweed (nori), and sliced into rounds. Sashimi is raw fish that is served with a dipping sauce. It is customary to eat sushi and sashimi together—but they are not the same food.

Some grocers sell sushi rolls premade and packaged in boxes, made at off-site locations. These vendors aren't the same ones who supply a prewrapped ham and cheese sandwich on a cold white roll; they specialize in Japanese cuisine. Though true sushi lovers say the quality suffers unless the rolls are made fresh and eaten immediately, the products are generally made from cooked ingredients, so they are no less safe than any other preprepared meal. Other stores go full out and have sushi chefs on-site who are trained in the rituals, traditions, and safety of preparing raw fish. These operations are also often franchised out to restaurants and catering companies that specialize in sushi and sashimi.

For raw fish, the quality and freshness can vary, but there is a good chance the supplier for a restaurant is the same as for an in-store sushi bar. There are only so many suppliers to go around. So, no matter where you buy sashimi, it most likely came from the same few sources. For instance, most yellowtail is farmed in Japan and comes from the same supplier, no matter where you partake of the delicacy.

Freshness is harder to pin down. Some top-of-the-line restaurants purchase their fish directly from Japan; however, most grocery store and restaurant sushi bars rely on import wholesalers who get their fish from various suppliers and on different days of the week. The transit can be overnight or take a few days. In general, Sunday and Monday are not good days to buy sashimi, because fish delivery companies take the weekend off.

Beyond the catch date, freshness is a tough call. The color and appearance won't tell you much. First, most sashimi- and sushi-grade fish is flash frozen to prevent parasites. Fish are frozen so quickly that water crystals never materialize, which is why the texture stays firm when thawed (unlike non-sushi-grade fish). Another trick is to gas raw tuna with carbon monoxide to prevent its rosy color from turning brown. If the fish is spoiled you won't know it until it's too late.

Here are some commonsense guidelines when buying sushi or sashimi at a grocery store (they apply to any restaurant as well):

1. Buy only sushi-grade fish; regular fish cannot be used to make sushi or sashimi because it is not flash frozen.

2. Find out the delivery dates. Do not buy sushi or sashimi on Sunday or even Monday. Most wholesalers do not make deliveries on the weekend.

3. Cleanliness counts. Make certain the sushi preparation counter and holding case are refrigerated and clean and the fish are not strewn about.

4. Fresh tuna will be red, but not too dark or too red. If it looks like lipstick red, it might be gassed with carbon monoxide.

5. If purchasing premade sushi rolls in a box, read the made date and/or sell-by date. Make certain the packages are stacked no more than two high, or they will most likely not be chilled well enough.

(continued)

6. Often fish used for sashimi is of higher quality than the specimens used for spicy tuna rolls because the ingredients mask flavor flaws.

7. Be aware of mercury levels. Recent studies show that 75% of sushi tuna samples taken from restaurants exceeded the EPA's safety limit—meaning pregnant women should probably avoid the stuff.

CHAPTER 6

Dairy Daze

Got rGBH-free Milk? Got Lawsuits

Imagine this question on a standardized high school test:

Peaceful Valley Dairy wants to label its milk so consumers know that no artificial growth hormones are injected into the cows to stimulate milk production. The FDA allows such labeling, provided the label does not mislead the consumer. Which one of the statements is more misleading?

(A) *Our Farmers' Pledge: No Artificial Growth Hormones*

(B) *Our Farmers' Pledge: No Artificial Growth Hormone Used*

(C) *None of the above*

It's not a trick question and it might be amusing, unless you are Oakhurst Dairy in Portland, Maine. The Bennett family, third-generation dairy owners, has supported the local 4-H dairy show, the town ticker-tape parade for returning veterans from Iraq, and a Little League baseball team. In 2003, Monsanto sued the dairy for deceiving consumers by labeling their products with statement (A).

Monsanto, maker of an artificial bovine growth hormone (rGBH) that stimulates milk production, based their case on the premise that statement (A) led consumers to believe that milk produced without the hormone is better than milk produced with the hormone. Other dairies had gone so far as to say. "No Hormones," which *is* misleading since all animal products contain naturally occurring hormones (the FDA cracked down on these labels). But Oakhurst's label made no such claim.

The "little dairy that could" eventually settled out of court with the corporate behemoth. Both agreed that label (B) was suitable, along with the disclaimer: *"FDA states: No significant difference in milk from cows treated with artificial growth hormones."* But basically, after all the lawyers and public-relations staff tallied their cut, it all came down to one word, "Used." According to *Webster's* (tenth ed.), the word has so many implications well suited to such a ridiculous case . . . old, worn, manipulated, consumed . . .

Outside of keeping the lawyers in business, the true underlying problem with rGBH is a clash between consumer perception and corporate muscle. Even if the milk composition is nearly identical, the word "hormone" has a negative connotation among milk drinkers. Even Monsanto refrains from the "H" word, now referring to the hormone by its synthetic name, recombinant Bovine Somatotropin (rBST). As if to say that consumers are bungling fools when buying our own food, the company apparently fails to see the issue is one of consumer preferance—not necessarily scientific weight.

It's hard to say how many dairies use the hormone; estimates vary from 15 to 30%. What is most disconcerting to wary milk drinkers is that milk from treated cows is pooled with milk from untreated cows. For consumers who prefer milk produced without the hormone, the only way to know the difference is through labeling—which to date has been an expensive and frustrating struggle.

Consumer interest groups have called for more studies to disprove the contention that the hormone doesn't have secondary effects, such as increased levels of IGF-1 (insulin-like growth factor) in milk and higher rates of antibiotic use.

Studies to date show IGF-1 levels may be higher in milk from treated cows; Monsanto says the increase is insignificant (which has been confirmed in more than one study). Clouding the issue is a theory that the hormone IGF-1, which assists in cell division in cows *and* humans, is higher in people diagnosed with colon, breast, lung, and prostate cancer. It is *not clear* that milk from cows treated with hormones plays a role in this.

As scientists delve further into whether rGBH-treated milk is truly identical to nontreated milk, the only peculiar fact is that IGF-1 survives the pasteurization process and when combined with casein (a milk protein) survives through the human gut. It is *not clear* whether this has any illness-causing implications, though a study in *The Journal of Reproductive Medicine* does speculate that bovine growth hormone may increase ovulation in women, which could increase the possibility of having twins. Whether this is construed as a negative result of rGBH in milk depends on your gender and your diaper and child-care budget. The International Dairy Council statement about the research underlines that this is theoretical and far from proven. As one can perfectly see, it is all speculative and not clear-cut. I hope *this is clear*.

What is known and recognized by an FDA warning on the drug's label is a side effect for increased rates of mastitis (udder infection), which can raise levels of—dare I say it—pus in milk. This sets up a cycle of extra antibiotic use, which in time may contribute to antibiotic resistance. Now before you let a pus and antibiotic fixation stop you from drinking milk, cows given antibiotics must be separated from the herd and all milk is tested for such impurities. In 2003, out of 3.5 million gallons of milk, less than .1% (.067%) tested positive for violating drug residue limits, including antibiotics. All milk that doesn't meet federal standards is thrown away. In all, mastitis costs the dairy industry as much as $2 billion a year in animal and milk production losses—why farmers would choose to use a drug that exacerbates this problem is not apparent.

One such group that supports the use of bovine growth hormones is the Center for Global Food Issues (a division of the Hudson Institute, which is supported by a broad array of companies and foundations not normally seen as supporting the same causes, such as the Pew Charitable Trusts and Monsanto). Although the group has vocally opposed any labeling of rGBH-free milk through its Web site, Stop Labeling Lies, they, too, developed a label, called Earth Friendly, Farm Friendly. I suppose it was a case of "if you can't beat 'em, join 'em."

When I called Alex Avery, the organization's leader, as well as author of a book, *The Truth About Organic Foods,* I expected an unpleasant conversation. This man and his father, Dennis Avery, are seen by some as the equivalent of Lex Luthor for the organic food industry. For decades, organic policy makers and the Center for Global Food Issues have argued through blog battles, scathing press releases, and public statements about the respective hazards and merits of genetically modified foods and bovine growth hormones.

After all the years of reading about the infamous father-son duo, I began with trepidation. After a few minutes of conversation . . . I have to admit that I actually liked the guy. We talked about schools for our children, book writing, our common interest in IPM-grown food (see the produce chapter), and even organic food—he likes chewy, crusty artisanal organic bread. It was very therapeutic, like a cleansing breath at a yoga class. OK, maybe not.

I digress. In between the *kumbaya* moments, we talked about his dairy label—more specifically, the failure of the Earth Friendly label. Apparently, no farmer was brave enough to stamp the symbol on their product, namely because one of the farming practices approved for certification was, you guessed it, bovine growth hormone. Certification required farmers to boost milk production using any two methods including breed selection, frequent milking, grass foraging, rotational grazing (all standard practices), and/or bovine growth hormone. Avery said that although he hasn't completely given up on the idea, the farmers are "afraid of getting sniped."

While Avery and I may be a bit like the food industry's version of Hannity and Colmes, we do agree that the hostility has grown to such a degree that farmers on both sides of the issue are afraid of snipers. Just as Avery's farming constituents aren't willing to fess up about using the hormone, neither are farmers who choose to abstain. Few are willing to hang in as long as Oakhurst Dairy. A recent tactic is to opt out of the hormone, though not label products accordingly. Case in point: The board of directors for Tillamook brand cheese in Oregon announced in 2005 that they would stop accepting milk from their cooperative dairies using the hormone. However, they will not label the products, to avoid the same litigious consequences as Oakhurst Dairy. Interested consumers will instead have to inquire.

The Milk and Cookie Conflict

Every Friday morning glass bottles of fresh, cold Colorado milk are delivered to my front door from the Longmont Dairy. It is nostalgic, it is local, it is not treated with artificial growth hormones, and it is pure luxury to pour off the cream into my morning cup of coffee.

The only thing my milk is not is organic, which is an anomaly in this region. The county where I reside is home to the corporate offices of the happy cow, Horizon Organic Dairy. The company founders had bigger dreams than home delivery. The once-small yogurt company is the largest organic dairy producer in the country, with an estimated 55% of the market share. Furthering their stature in the market, Horizon was bought by Dean Foods—the largest conventional dairy company in the nation.

Now that Dean Foods supplies stores like Wal-Mart with organic milk, critics say the principles of organic food production are turning sour. I call the controversy the Milk and Cookie Conflict. At the top of the organic shopping list for megastores, like Wal-Mart, are entry-level products like organic milk and cookies; the sales growth for both exceeds 20%. The deliriously fast pace has led some to believe that the milk can't possibly be organic enough or that packaged foods must be made from only the purest ingredients, with no give for the constraints of commercial food production (read more about cookies in the packaged foods chapter).

Critics, the half-empty milk glass assembly, are disgruntled because they believe this high demand is forcing large organic dairies to cut corners. Leading the charge is the Cornucopia Institute, whose motto is: "Promoting Economic Justice for Family-Scale Farming." To drive their position to the forefront, Cornucopia published a grading report of organic dairy farms called *Maintaining the Integrity of Organic Milk*.

Since the mid-1900s Mark Kastel, cofounder of Cornucopia, has been fighting against what he calls the industrialization of the organic industry and large-scale farms that barely meet the spirit of the organic rules. Now that the USDA oversees the organic certification process, getting opinions heard, noticed, and followed is even more difficult.

The group has targeted their frustration on two fronts. In addition to a filing a lawsuit against the USDA to gain access to documents regarding organic policy making, they have targeted two companies, Horizon Organic Dairy and Aurora Organic Dairy, calling them no better than factory farms. These are *fightin'* words. "Factory farming" is perhaps the most blasphemous term possible in the organic food world.

Horizon's happy-cow headquarters is a few miles south of my front door; their largest dairy is near Twin Falls, Idaho. The remaining farms are large and small contracted farms across the country. Aurora, a private label supplier, is just across town to the north; they also own a large dairy farm in Texas and recently opened another farm here in Colorado. These two companies, which are holding much of the fortuitous overspill of soaring consumer demand for organic milk, are accused by Cornucopia of many small transgressions, but the most visible is bypassing a requirement for pasturing animals and creating farms of gargantuan proportions, with more than 3,000 cows per herd.

Despite what one may think, organic certification for all types of farms does not mandate size—any size farm can be certified organic. The discrepancies lie in the NOP guidelines, which say livestock must have access to the outdoors and direct sunlight and the conditions must be "suitable to the species, its stage of production, the climate and environment." The animals must have "access to pasture for ruminants," but the rules do not specify how much pasture or how long the cows should be in a pasture.

These two companies interpret the rules in this way: Aurora Dairy feeds cows with certified-organic cut grass and grains in bunks (troughs), while the cows wait for their milking in shaded sheds or pasture, depending on the season. Horizon provides pasture space as well as certified-organic cut grass and grains in bunks. Both are adding more pasture space to their largest dairies in the coming year. (See the Addendum in the back for an update.) The claim from Kastel is that with each farm's current farming conditions, these megafarms could never be licensed as organic without exerting undue influence on certifiers. Worse yet, the report accused the dairies of pandering to the cost-cutting measures of Wal-Mart, in order to supply such megabox stores with cheap organic milk.

These are pretty serious accusations, so much so that the Organic Consumer's Union, a consumer activist group, not associated with Cornucopia, asked consumers and retailers to boycott Horizon Dairy products. The appeal reached zealous co-ops and health-food store retailers across the country, and many immediately pulled the milk from the shelves. Aurora's private label status offered some protection from the boycott, since it sells to grocery-store private label brands.

Cornucopia calls the report a guide to allow consumers to easily spot "organic dairy products produced with the best organic practices." Should consumers boycott these dairies and use the report as organic gospel? If consumers west of the Rockies and in the Southwest use this report as a so-called *guide,* there are very few dairies to choose from. Of the sixty-eight reviewed brands, only one dairy with distribution in the Rocky Mountain region received a favorable grade. For California shoppers, only one small dairy, with limited distribution, got a good rating.

Suspicious? The survey was voluntary. Eastern- and Northern-based dairies that participated were graded favorably. Most Western dairies were judged based on "industry sources," none receiving higher than a "questionable commitment to organic." Cornucopia defends publication of the report, saying it was never meant to be scientific but instead a scorecard to "showcase ethical family farms and expose factory farm producers and brands that threaten to take over organic dairying."

In this Westerner's opinion, the report fails to mention that much of the quarrel comes down to the most fought over fluid natural resource in the history of man—not oil, certainly not milk; think water. It's hard to fathom, especially for visitors who perhaps ski over Colorado's 300 inches of packed powder or fly-fish in our mountain streams, but much of the region is dry and arid.

Case in point: The rainfall in my town, Longmont, the closest municipality to the most vilified organic "factory farm," Aurora Dairy, is 13.9 inches—that's per year—as compared to more than 40 inches in the Northeast. A wide expanse of land, but no water, paints a very different picture of organic farming than that in other regions with acres of water and postage-stamp-size farms.

The organic rules are meant to recognize this polarity and allow for variations in farming practices. Here are a few examples of how farms across the country differ: A small Eastern dairy may be home to as few as 50 to 100 cows because the farm's size is locked in by centuries-old zoning restrictions, while a *small* Western dairy farmer may own as many as 300 to 500 cows and have hundreds more acres to expand. Both farms are considered *small* organic dairies. Also, an Eastern organic dairy farmer may seldom allow the cows out of the barn in the winter because of harsh conditions. In the West, though, a dairy may let its cows roam about in the winter sun. Both farms are still *small* organic dairies.

Organic dairies with more than 3,000 cows have been criticized for not having enough or any pasture grass available. As a consumer, do I really care whether cows pull every tuft of grass they eat from the ground or eat dried certified organic grass from troughs? It's a toss-up. No matter whether the feed grows on-site or elsewhere, it's still organically grown. If the organic laws require a specific square footage for pasture, then certainly dairies should follow the standards, but to date this isn't required. Honestly, when city lawmakers tell me I could be fined for watering my vegetable garden on the wrong day, I'd rather see farmers be equally restrained with their water use, since 80% of the water is used for agriculture. Honestly, water conservation means more to me than milk boycotts.

Recent weather patterns illustrate the dilemma. In the very same month the National Organic Standards board met to review pasturing rules for organic dairies, the Northeast was drenched with destructive floods, of one-hundred-year proportions, while in the West irrigation wells in Colorado's eastern plains were shut down for lack of water because of an ongoing six-year drought. Governors on both sides of the country called states of emergencies, each for very different reasons.

Are large-scale dairies the epitome of Upton Sinclair's *The Jungle,* the very "killing beds" Jurgis worked in to support Ona, his new bride? Worse yet, are the corporate interests of big-box stores shutting out the interests of the small farmer? Hardly. In fact, small dairy farmers who contract with these so-called industrialized corporate dairy companies say for the first time in many years they can pay bills and support their families, because organic dairy sales are so strong and the income is steady.

In truth, only four farms in the entire organic dairy industry could be categorized as large-scale, as opposed to 15% of conventional dairies in the West that are larger than 1,000 head. The Cornucopia report failed to mention that Horizon contracts with as many as 325 small family farms from coast to coast.

Aurora supports nearly two hundred small farms that grow organic feed and provide pasture space. Perhaps the most damning accusation from Cornucopia directed at Aurora is a photograph of the farm displayed prominently on its Web site, which was picked up by many newspapers across the nation. The photograph features an overhead shot of a brown swath of land used as milking pens. The caption says, "Aurora 'organic' factory confinement dairy—Platteville, Colorado."

The photograph has been cropped down so small that it cuts out the hundreds of surrounding acres of organic pasture that the company contracts from small local farmers. In addition, since the processing plant is on site (which is also cropped out of the photograph), there are virtually no transportation emissions. The company refers to it as from "Cow to Carton."

Since none of these facts ever emerged in the dozens of newspaper reports, zealous grocers called for organic dairy boycotts from Portland, Maine, to Portland, Oregon—a move that could have placed hundreds of small organic dairies across the country in jeopardy. It's lucky that since organic milk is so undersupplied, by as much as 20%, with demand climbing by the same percentage each year, the affected dairies barely noticed the boycotts. It is estimated that our farming system would have to add 100,000 more organic dairy cows just to keep up with the current demand.

What Cornucopia really wants is a higher standard of organic than the rules demand. They are looking for a farming ethic that embodies concepts like small farm size and no imported grain. Even though as of this writing no inspector can find any examples of animal cruelty on any of the so-called "factory farms," Cornucopia says that it's impossible for the cows to be treated well on such large operations. The institute is calling for USDA to define exact scale parameters for organic dairies. And even though each company offers benefits that few small farms can provide, such as well-paying salaries, 401k plans, profit sharing, and health benefits, Kastel said in an interview he wants the organic certification to include social ethic and fair wages for organic farm workers. It's doubtful that these ideologies will ever become public policy, since the USDA certifies organic dairies and takes no sides in social ethos. Farmers who employ these qualities are welcome to market their products as such or conceivably Cornucopia will have to come up with their own third-party certification that meets Kastel's standards.

Cornucopia got the attention it desired. Major media outlets around the nation that had never heard of Cornucopia picked up the story. Kastel was pleased with the "flames of controversy" the report generated. A few months after Cornucopia's report, the pasture requirements for organic dairies were reexamined and a guidance document was presented to the USDA that called for cows to get one-third of their food directly from pastures. It is too soon to tell if any permanent changes will occur. In the meantime, Horizon added more pasture space—Kastel complained to USDA that it wasn't adequate. Aurora decided to decrease the number of cows to 1,000 on its much-publicized Platteville, Colorado, location and move the remaining cows farther north to a newly built grassy farm. But at the same time, Kastel is still in the half-empty glass assembly, believing that nothing monumental will come about, which means he will most likely find fault with other sectors of organic farming and get the word out.

My hunch is that even if changes are mandated, the dairies in question will never look like the utopian rain-soaked models of the North and East. Kastel has suggested that organic dairy production be restricted to regions that can offer more naturally growing grass with less irrigation than our parched climate. This assertion means that Western consumers would be held hostage to dairies as far away as Wisconsin or New Hampshire purely to meet the unreasonable expectations of others. Trucking organic milk across the country hardly seems ecologically sound. Sadly, the meddling only pits farmers against one another about who is a better steward of organic farming.

Dairy Labeling

TYPES OF FLUID MILK

In 1999, milk labeling changed from words like "skim" and "low fat" to a host of new possibilities like "2%, reduced fat" and "1%, low fat." One might assume that the label means that 2% of the fat was removed or 2g of fat remain. What it really means is the milk contains 2% fat by weight, which is about half the fat of whole milk. The same applies for low-fat milk, which contains 1% fat by weight, which is about one-quarter the fat of whole milk. Here is a side-by-side comparison of the fat content for each type:

Name	Total Fat (one cup)	% Daily Value (2,000-cal. diet)	Calories (one cup)
Whole Milk	8 g	12%	150
Reduced Fat, Less Fat, 2%	4.7 g	7%	122
Low Fat, 1%	2.6 g	4%	102
Skim, Fat Free, Nonfat	>.5 g	0%	80

Pasteurized Milk   Milk is highly perishable and under poorly supervised conditions bacteria can quickly contaminate milk, which is why pasteurization is called for. Before it was mandatory, my great-grandmother, a Michigan dairy farmer's wife, heated milk from her farm before letting my father take even a sip. Disease experts call pasteurization one of the greatest food safety accomplishments of our time. Today there are small pockets of resistance to this widely used practice.

One hub of support for this practice is in a community just north of my home, Guidestone Farms, in Loveland, Colorado. David Lynch, owner of the farm, and his supporters (Campaign for Real Milk) convinced the Colorado Board of Health to allow customers to buy shares of a dairy cow, as one would purchase stock in a company. As partial owners, the "stockholders" get to keep the dividends. In this case, the payout is unpasteurized raw milk.

The Campaign for Real Milk believes that pasteurized milk is "adulterated" because of enzyme destruction, protein alterations, homogenization, synthetic vitamin fortification, and vitamin destruction. Proponents of raw milk insist that proper cleanliness overcomes any risk from potential spread of bacteria. Opponents say even under the cleanest conditions there is a risk to health, especially for pregnant women and children. More than a few cases of *E. coli* and salmonella are reported each year from raw milk consumption.

Raw milk followers would like to see a recognized inspection system for raw milk to ensure cleanliness and purity. For small farms with limited distribution, this may be possible. Based on the current statistics for food-borne outbreaks for foods like produce, poultry, and beef, there is no certainty, though, that the already overworked and underfunded agricultural inspection system could ever support such a plan. Stand by.

Ultrapasteurized Milk and Cream   With the exception of raw milk, all milk, organic or otherwise, is pasteurized. There is an additional process that heats milk and cream to 280 degrees, called ultra-high-temperature (UHT) pasteurization, which kills bacteria and extends shelf life to months, rather then weeks. Whipping cream and half-and-half are often sold with UHT pasteurization because the turnover isn't as high as that for fluid milk.

More recently some organic milk suppliers have resorted to UHT pasteurization because they have to ship milk farther away to keep up with growing demand. Few realize that the unopened expiration date on their milk is fifty days away when ordinarily it would be a week or two. When supplies outstripped demand, many organic milk companies began using UHT pasteurization to prevent spoilage.

The biggest victim of UHT pasteurization is taste—ultrapasteurized milk tastes like cooked milk. The only indicator of ultrapasteurized milk is on the ingredient list or nutrition panel. Even with these precautions, remember that once opened, all milk and cream, UHT or not, lasts only about one week. So even though that lovely organic milk you buy may say it will hold unopened for fifty days, once you break the seal it has the same seven-day life span as any other type of milk or cream.

ECO-FRIENDLY LABELS

USDA Organic Certified   As seen earlier, the organic certification standards regarding organic milk production are evolving. Even so, the organic seal means that a minimum of standards is met. Organically certified cows are not given antibiotics, exposed to pesticides, or injected with growth hormones. Once certified, the feed is 100% organic. In addition to worries about vague pasture requirements, there are concerns about loopholes that allow for use of 20% nonorganic feed during a conventional cow's transition to organic.

Even with a resolution of these issues, understand that the organic rules allow farmers to decide how to best care for their animals based on the conditions of their respective regions. Neither is any more or less organic than the other. As a consumer, if you prefer Cornucopia's definition of "organic," there are plenty of dairies to choose from, and if you are fine with letting the farmer decide how best to satisfy the organic standards, these brands are available at all types of stores.

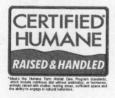

Certified Humane   This program is overseen by the Humane Farm Animal Care. USDA certified the inspectors to make certain that bovine growth hormones are prohibited and the animals are raised on a diet free of animal by-products. The animals must be raised with adequate space and in a manner that allows natural behaviors.

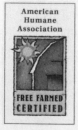

Free Farmed   These dairy cows are certified by the AHA. The association's certification process for livestock monitors the conditions for food, water, shelter, and grazing space. The certification process forbids the use of growth hormones and animal by-products in feed.

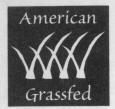

Grass-Fed   Grass-fed cows graze in pastures for most, if not all, of their producing lives. They are not fed grain, ever. The American Grassfed Association is hoping for a USDA-approved certification program in the future. The health advantage of grass-fed milk is that it is higher in vitamin A, vitamin E, omega-3 fatty acids, and CLA. It is believed that these healthy fatty acids have been depleted from our food supply over time as farming methods moved from grazing to mostly corn feed.

DAIRY CASE HEALTH CLAIMS

We need calcium and vitamin D to build bones; there is no getting around it. One cup of dairy is an easy way to get 300mg of calcium; however, there are options if you can't eat dairy or prefer to avoid it. The easiest means are dairy alternatives like soy, rice, and nut milks, which are fortified with calcium and vitamin D. The following are FDA-approved health claims for dairy and nondairy alternatives:

Calcium and Osteoporosis
A diet adequate in calcium may help reduce the risk for osteoporosis, a degenerative bone disease.

The product must contain 20% or more of the 200mg Daily Value (DV) for calcium per serving and contain a form of calcium that is easily absorbed by the body.

When you see an important nutrient, such as calcium, on the label, know how to read the percentage value. For instance, if the nutrition panel on a dairy product says "15%," this means one serving will provide 15% of the total amount one needs for the entire day. Calcium percentages are fairly standard from one brand of milk to another; however, they can vary from one brand of yogurt to another.

Soy Protein and Coronary Heart Disease
Diets low in saturated fat and cholesterol that include 25g of soy protein a day may reduce the risk of heart disease. One serving of [name of food] provides _____ grams of soy protein.

Soy beverages with this health claim must be low fat (3g or less), low saturated fat (1g or less), and low cholesterol (20mg or less). Soy beverages are fortified to contain as much as or more calcium than milk. A word of sweet caution, though: Soy beverages often have high amounts of added sugar or corn syrup to soften the bean taste.

DAIRY WITH CULTURE

It was my job as a child to turn the jars of milk in my Greek grandparents' basement. With the right twist of the wrist and enough warm blankets, milk would turn to yogurt. Greeks have long treasured the health properties of yogurt. It all comes down to microbes that digest milk sugars called lactose. This process forms dozens of helpful microbes that inhibit the formation of harmful bacteria, especially in the gut.

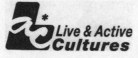 Here are three considerations when purchasing yogurt: First, you want live active cultures; second, you want a variety of living cultures; and third, remember that some products are loaded with sugar, which is counter to a seemingly healthy product.

Not all yogurts are as cultured as others. They all start out that way, but heat processes destroy the helpful bacteria. Look for some assurance that the product has a preponderance of live cultures. You may see numbers like 10^{10}, which mathematically means billions and billions of active cultures. The National Yogurt Association (NYA) seal is a guarantee that the cultures are alive. To qualify for the seal the company must have testing verification from a state- or USDA-approved laboratory. As important, look for Latin words that resemble the names of Greek tragedy actors. The most common are *lactobacillus acidophilus, lactobacillus bulgaricus,* and *streptococcus thermophilus.* More recent discoveries include *lactobacillus casei, bifidobacterium bifidum, lactobacillus reuteri,* and *lactobacillus plantarum.*

If my grandfather were still alive today, he would question whether the yogurt in today's grocery case is the same dairy food he made in the basement. The most he might have added to plain yogurt was a teaspoon of honey or jam, but today's commercial brands can be loaded with sugar or corn syrup.

Unfortunately, our labeling laws don't distinguish between naturally occurring sugars and added sugars. So for instance, a six-ounce carton of plain yogurt has 11g of naturally occurring milk sugars. You will have to memorize this number to know how much added sweetener is in a standard six-ounce container of strawberry yogurt. The label might say as much as 44g sugar; subtract the 11g of milk sugar, which leaves 33g. At 4g of sugar or high-fructose corn syrup per teaspoon, that six-ounce strawberry yogurt has a little more than eight teaspoons of sweetener. Yes, that's eight teaspoons in a tiny six-ounce cup, so watch out.

Prebiotics are the latest additive to enhance the health properties of yogurt. The most commonly used prebiotic in foods is inulin, a fiber that gels in the stomach. It's one of the many fermented fibers that help boost the amount of beneficial gut bacteria. Prebiotics also slow down your digestion. This gives the body more time to take in minerals like calcium, iron, and magnesium, which increases bioavailability by as much as 38%. These coagulating wonder fibers may also play a role in fighting colon cancer by reducing the amount of harmful pathogens in the colon. Look for inulin in the ingredients or a statement like "with FOS," which is short for fructooligosaccharides, a type of inulin.

TRANS FAT LABELS

Ever since the Parkay margarine tub posed the question, "Butter or Margarine?" consumers have been confused as to what to buy. Culinary gastronomists say butter, but cardiologists prefer that we turn to liquid fats such as extra-virgin olive oil (EVOO), nut oils, and canola oil. If necessary use tub margarine, but only if it is truly free of trans fats, also called partially hydrogenated fats.

Naturally occurring trans fats are produced in small quantities in the guts of all ruminant animals, from cows to camels. As a result, we get small amounts of trans fats from butter, dairy, and meat. The other type of trans fat is manufactured by turning a liquid oil into a solid by "partially saturating" the fat with hydrogen molecules (hence the name partially hydrogenated fats). Add some water, flavoring, and a bit more oil to the mix and you've got margarine.

Like saturated fats, trans fats can raise lipid cholesterols (low-density lipoprotein or LDL), but trans fats also decrease HDL (high-density lipoprotein), the healthy cholesterol that rids the blood of unhealthy fats. Cardiologists recommend margarines made with no trans fats and brands with plant sterols and plant stanols, bioactive additives that can reduce cholesterol levels.

Don't be misled by margarine labels that say "No trans fat, per serving." These products still contain heart-damaging trans fats; however, because the serving size is small the manufacturer may make the claim. Any product that contains .5g or less of trans fats per serving is by law allowed to say, "No trans fat, per serving." For assurance, check the ingredient panel to make certain there are no hydrogenated fats, such as hydrogenated soybean or canola oil, listed in the ingredients.

Cheese Labels

The labeling laws for European cheeses are well entrenched in food law, none perhaps more than those for Parmigiano-Reggiano. Muscular men from Parma, dressed in white aprons and cream-colored rubber boots, fill copper vats with milk each morning. With the precision of chemists, they heat and stir the milk until curds form. With the strength of weight lifters, they hoist the eighty-pound wheels into linen blankets for curing. Each wheel will be checked and rechecked during the one–three year aging process. Only the cheese that meets the strict standards will bear the quality seal stamped on the outer rind of the cheese and the name Parmigiano-Reggiano.

Other cheese makers have tried to use the name Parmigiano, Parmesan, and dozens of other colloquialisms. By E.U. law unless the cheese is made in a specific region near Parma, with approved farming methods and just the right cows, the cheese cannot bear the name Parmigiano-Reggiano or even Parmesan. Since 2002, imposter "Parmesan" cheese makers in the E.U. have turned to their dictionaries and marketing experts to come up with new names. It doesn't roll off the tongue as nicely as Parmigiano, but the most popular wording so far is "Italian grated cheese." The E.U. food courts also ruled in favor of

"Greek feta," noting the cheese has been made since Homer's *Odyssey,* even though Denmark makes more of it than Greece.

So what impact does this have on a country that invented plastic-wrapped singles and cheese in a squirt can? While protesters took to the streets about poverty, tariffs, and farm subsidies at the 2005 World Trade talks in Cancun, American cheese makers waited to hear whether they might have to rename their products. The E.U. has a list of forty-one different food product names it would like to protect, such as Comte and Roquefort cheese from France, Manchego cheese from Spain, and mozzarella and Gorgonzola from Italy. The decision never came to the forefront, so the fate is uncertain for the pulverized cheese in the squirt can or, for that matter, mozzarella made in Texas or Gouda made in Wisconsin. There must be something in the Declaration of Independence that allows explicit freedom to name any yellow block cheese in the colonies "cheddar." But who knows, maybe the British are coming to reclaim their birthright to cheddar?

COMMERCIAL CHEESE

While specialty cheese ages for years in dank cellars, commercial block cheese might be aged for a whisper of time, a few months, or more than a year. The longer cheese ages, the sharper the taste. The most popular commercial cheeses in America are the Fab Four: cheddar, Colby, Monterey Jack, and Swiss. They are aged in plastic vacuum wrapping, cut, and repackaged in plastic or wax for individual sale.

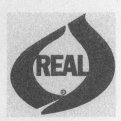

The United Dairy Industry Association marks milk and cheese with this "REAL" seal if the product is made from U.S.-produced milk and the product does not contain oils, casein, or fillers—in other words, no imitation cheese is allowed. Look for it on dairy products and frozen pizza. The most popular commercial cheeses in America are the following.

Cheddar   The name "cheddar" comes from a region in England, as well as a process used to make cheddar cheese. "Cheddaring" means the cheese curds are stacked and matted together until they form slabs. The slabs are stacked and turned for about two hours.

Cheddar is labeled with aging characteristics of mild, medium, and sharp (aged). Mild ages from a mere ten days to four months; medium ages four to ten months; aged and sharp wait from about ten months to a few years.

Colby This yellow block cheese looks like cheddar, but it is made without the traditional "cheddaring" process. The texture is moist and soft, and this cheese has less sodium than cheddar.

Monterey Jack This American invention is named for Monterey, California, where the cheese originated, and the last name of the man who marketed it, David Jacks. Traditional Monterey Jack cheese isn't aged; there are, however, new brands of aged Monterey Jack, called Dry Jack, that are worth trying.

Swiss Commercially made Swiss without rinds is an American invention, one that uses pressure plates to form the cheese. The holes form during the three-to-four-month aging process from a culture that is added to the milk. The culture gives Swiss cheese a sweet nutty flavor and helps form carbon dioxide that creates air bubbles in the cheese.

TYPES OF ARTISANAL CHEESE
Now that artisanal cheeses are better appreciated in this country, supermarket cases are a bit cramped and are a good lesson in the Romance languages. Most retailers separate artisanal and specialty cheeses from commercial or deli cheese, but it can be difficult to know what's what. Here is a synopsis of what you may find.

Fresh Soft Cheese This cheese is made from the first stage of cheese making. It is unripened, spreadable, and perishable. It should be purchased as close to the date you plan to eat it as possible. Examples: cream cheese, cottage cheese, farmer's cheese, fromage blanc, fresh goat cheese, soft herbed cheese, mascarpone, mizithra, paneer, ricotta, and queso fresco or blanco.

Soft Cheese   These cheeses ripen for a short time, giving them a pliable, downy rind and smooth interior. Examples: Brie, Brillat Savarin, Camembert, aged goat, ricotta salata, St. Andre.

Brine-Packed Cheese   As these cheeses dry out quickly, they are packed in a protected liquid bath. Examples: feta, fresh mozzarella, and teleme.

Stretched Curd Cheese   This cheese gets its stringy texture from stretching and kneading when the cheese is warm (called *pasta filata*). The cheese used to be pulled and knotted exclusively by hand. Though there are still some exceptions, it's mostly pulled by machines today. American cheese making has taken this essential step out of domestic provolone, so the flavors will vary among domestic and imported brands. Examples: aged mozzarella, imported provolone, caciocavallo (pronounced "kachio-ka-VA-lo") cheese.

Blue Cheese   These cheeses are made by adding mold to the curds or inoculating the cheese with spores. Examples: blue cheese, Roquefort, Gorgonzola, Stilton.

Washed-Rind Cheese   This type of cheese ripens from the outside in, under very humid conditions. The rind has a characteristic reddish-brown color. Examples: Appenzeller, Brick, Limburger, Morbier, Taleggio.

Semifirm Cheese   Pressing during aging gives these cheeses a soft, pliable texture, good for slicing and sandwiches. Examples: Asiago, cheddar, Comte, Edam, Emmentaler, Fontina, Gruyère, Jarlsberg, Manchego, Swiss.

Hard Cheese   This cheese is known for robust, deep flavors and long shelf life. The texture is perfectly suited for grating and breaking off into chunks. Hard cheese, such as Parmigiano-Reggiano, is speckled with shiny crystals; these are amino acids that give the cheese a crunchy texture. Many semifirm cheeses can be aged into a hard cheese. Examples: Dry Jack, Grana Padano, Kefalotyri, Parmigiano-Reggiano, Pecorino, queso enchilada, Romano.

CHEESE WHIZARDS

Even the time-honored world of cheese making isn't exempt from American ingenuity, as witnessed by the number of processed cheese products, cold pack, grated, reduced-fat, and functional food cheeses. Each of these types of cheese is defined by USDA guidelines. For better or worse, there are some creative cheesy inventions in the dairy case.

Pasteurized Process Cheese This product is made by grinding and blending, with the aid of heat and an emulsifying agent, one or more natural cheeses into a "homogeneous mass." Cheese food has added ingredients like cream, milk, nonfat milk, buttermilk, cheese whey, anhydrous milk fat, dehydrated cream, or skim milk cheese. Other optional ingredients include emulsifying agents, acidifying agents, water, salt, artificial coloring, and spices and flavorings.

Grated Cheese The name is self-explanatory, except the manufacturer is allowed to make a few changes, including reducing the moisture content and adding mold-inhibiting and anticaking ingredients. If you've ever wondered about that fine powder that coats grated cheese, it's a dusting of plant fibers to prevent sticking. Often these additives change the way the cheese melts—you may have better results for cheese sauces if you start with block cheese instead of pregrated.

Reduced-Fat Cheese To make cheese, a certain amount of fat is needed for the necessary reactions to occur. This requisite adds a certain degree of difficulty to reduced-fat cheese making. Something has to give in the process, and it's usually texture and flavor. For consumers with medical reasons to eat low-fat products, these products are useful, despite the flavor and texture changes. Recipe developers find that 50% reduced-fat cheeses work well in recipes.

Plant Sterols In 2000, a health claim was approved for plant sterols and stanols, citing their ability to reduce cholesterol. Since then food scientists have worked to find ways to use them in food. They need fat for solubility, so sterols and stanols are well suited as additives for cheese, salad dressings, and margarine. To see a noticeable difference in cholesterol levels, though, you must consume two portions per day. Reduced-fat cheeses are the only types of cheese that qualify for the plant-sterol health claim.

Bottom Line

As the granddaughter of Greek emigrants, I was weaned on feta cheese, yogurt, and rice pudding in my high chair. No Kraft cheese or Jell-O pudding for this kid. As soon I was tall enough to reach the jukebox at my grandfather's diner in Detroit, the waitresses let me pick the song. Propped up at the counter at the Star Waffle Diner, I ate rice pudding and feta cheese and swung my legs to "Downtown" by Petula Clark while the waitresses danced with plates of fried eggs and hot coffee. It was pure unadulterated fun and the Michigan milk that was delivered through the back door each day was equally pure— no artificial growth hormones *used*.

Proponents of rGBH say consumer groups fighting to rid the dairy industry of the hormone are hiding behind other agendas like vegan and dairy-free diets. True, the most persistent and vocal groups may be attached to agendas that reach far beyond the dairy industry.

Nonetheless, consumers without such deep-seated convictions, who dance in diners, drink milk, and eat meat, are making their wishes known through the old-fashioned American dollar. These shoppers haven't the time or the interest to become activists, but they do want milk and cheese made without rGBH. For farmers meeting this demand, it's paying off. Commodity prices for milk constantly fall short of farmers' expectations, and conventional dairy sales are at best flat. Farmers brave enough to label their products with "No Artificial Hormones Used," and the like, have a competitive edge of as much as $1.50 extra per gallon. Organic prices are even higher.

It's sad that the organic dairy industry is falling into the same litigious overreactions as the bovine growth hormone supporters. The rules for organic certification came about because farmers of all types and policy makers of all ilks sat at the same table, regardless of their differences, and made decisions. Somehow this pluralism has eroded. The organic rules were meant to evolve; however, when retailers ask the consumers to take sides with boycotts, it will only serve to hurt farmers who are committed to organic agriculture.

It has been suggested that some regions of the country, like Texas and the arid West, should not produce organic milk, ever. Customers would instead have to rely on organic milk shipments from far and beyond. This hardly seems like a practical solution. Organic milk is so sought after that supply already falls short of demand. By the end of the week, organic dairy cases across the country are often empty—no happy cows, no organic valleys, not even private label brands. Some shoppers, with a shaky commitment to organic, will tire of this trend and return to conventional milk. Turning away from our own local organic farmers will only sour their success and our own regional farming economies.

CHAPTER 7

Grains of Truth: Pasta, Bread, Cereal, and Grains

Low-Carb Letdown

The French have a term for food window-shopping, "licking the windows." During our nation's low-carb craze as many as 30% of American dieters licked the windows of the pasta, grain, bread, and cereal aisles to satisfy their underserved carbohydrate cravings. The fervor was so passionate that I knew middle-aged women who gave up on lifelong friendships because they couldn't eat together. Their differences of opinion about low-carb diets were too big to overcome. Even the publishing company I was employed by came under pressure from our largest advertiser, Atkins Nutritionals, to create more low-carb recipes for readers. Our response was, until the advertisers signed our paychecks, we had no plans to change our editorial calendar.

That day never came. Atkins filed for bankruptcy on August 1, 2005, largely due to competition from other major food producers who joined in on the trend with hundreds of new low-carb products that flooded the market. Competition was the final chapter, though the company's bad luck started months earlier. A coroner's report showed signs of heart disease in the company's founder, Dr. Robert Atkins, after he died from a fall on an icy New York sidewalk in 2003. Atkins company officials tried to account for coroner's test results as postinjury weight gain from IV fluids and a past history of heart disease. But regardless of the cause of death, the mere speculation of heart disease was hardly the type of news millions of low-carb followers wanted to hear.

By 2005, America came out of its ketosis-induced fog and returned to the comfort of carbohydrates, but it wasn't like coming home. A host of new grain products entered the market, each one designed to compete with the hundreds of low-carb products. If any good came from the low-carb movement, the new foods emphasized the value of whole grains. Even white bread now has more fiber, whole-grain pasta isn't hidden in the health-food aisle, and whole-grain cereals offer some nutritional sanity to the sugar-laden cereal department.

Was the pasta ban justified? My Italian friends thought we Americans were *pazzo*, crazy, that pasta was written off as a forbidden food. If the same antipasta philosophy took over in Italy the entire economy would collapse. They were right to question our sanity.

One hard, fast rule of low-carbohydrate eating was no white food, namely, refined flours. Pasta is white, but it is not made from refined flour. Pasta is made from semolina flour (noodles are made from refined flour). Semolina is the endosperm, the nutrition-packed tip of the durum wheat kernel that feeds the plant's embryo. It's rich in protein at 8g per half-cup serving and has a modest amount of fiber (2g). Whole-wheat pasta blends further increase the fiber quotient with flaxseed, wheat bran, and germ, which add additional heart health benefits.

As always, it was the portion size, not the pasta, that got Americans into weight-gain trouble. Just what is one serving of pasta? The box suggests that two ounces is one serving. That's nice—but what does two ounces of long thin spaghetti look like? An easily recognizable gauge is a penny and a quarter. A penny will sit securely on the end of a two-ounce serving of thin spaghetti (when held tightly, an inch from the top); a quarter will do the same for a four-ounce serving. Two ounces of shaped pasta, such as penne or bow ties, is three-quarters of a cup of dried pasta.

The last gaffe that raised our blood sugar, and the blood pressure of Italians, was cooking time. Pasta must be cooked al dente to retain the nutritional properties and the taste of the semolina flour. Al dente, translated as cooked "to the tooth," pasta will leave a small white dot or band in the center of the pasta. The cooking times vary by the pasta shape and thickness, but in my experience, al dente cooking times can be one to two minutes shorter than the recommended cooking time on the box.

Pasta cooking times can also make a difference in your health. Researchers who study how foods impact blood sugar say that al dente–cooked pasta doesn't cause blood sugar to spike as does over-cooked, mushy pasta. Just watch your portions.

The Lowdown on Glycemic Index

One of the drawbacks to the low-carb craze was there was no single well-defined meaning for the term, which meant manufacturers could manipulate the data to suit their needs. Consumer Labs, a watchdog company for labeling claims on dietary supplements and functional foods, tested protein bars, energy bars, and meal replacement bars and found that many of the products were mislabeled for carbohydrates— one exceeded the values on the label by 33g.

A more accurate measure of carbohydrates may be a concept that has been around for nearly thirty years called the glycemic index (GI). The term may be new to your ears and food labels, but it's not new to physicians who treat diabetics. Doctors have long advised their diabetic patients to pay attention to low-glycemic foods, as defined by the GI, which measures individual foods—not entire categories like carbohydrates—for their impact on blood sugar.

The rudimentary version of low-carb fanaticism vilified all carbohydrates. The GI makes a clearer distinction because it measures exactly how one metabolizes specific foods and how fast and how far blood sugar rises from ingestion to digestion (called insulin response). Each food is assigned a clinical rating, a GI, based on the amount of insulin released in the bloodstream. Highly processed white bread owns the pinnacle of glycemic responses—it's 70–100, depending on how it is processed. The GI for whole-grain bread (made with a blend of whole wheat and barley) is knocked down to the midfifties, and so on, for hundreds of thousands of foods.

To drive the message home, pasta is often used as an example of how an ill-perceived food can be resurrected with GI ratings. Pasta, cooked al dente, has a relatively low GI ranking (41); overcooked pasta is considered high GI. Oats are another example—slow-cooked whole oats have a low GI ranking; quick-cooked oats have a high GI status. Proponents of the GI principle say that if the average person ingests too many high-GI foods, blood sugar rises and the excess is stored as fat around vital organs like the heart and liver, as well as abdominal fat—thus increasing the chances of developing type 2 diabetes and heart disease.

One of the most influential scientists for the GI cause is Dr. Ann de Wees Allen. I've never met her in person, but I think she is a brave soul. Dr. Allen is the chief of biomedical research at the Glycemic Research Institute in Washington, D.C. When the low-carb craze was at its height of popularity, Dr. Allen toured with Dr. Atkins at medical conferences and played devil's advocate to the popular diet guru. Even with the fanaticism surrounding Atkins, Allen held her ground that high-fat, high-protein diets were not healthy and could easily lead to high blood pressure, kidney stones, osteoporosis, and increased risk of heart disease and cancer.

Dr. Allen's belief is that the Atkins diet plan went astray because of the misconception that the body could function properly on 30g or less of carbohydrates per day and all that butter, meat, and cream wouldn't take its ultimate toll on the human heart. She knows her advice sounds a lot like your mother's, but the human body functions best on mostly fruits, vegetables, whole grains, and lean proteins. Dr. Allen says the healthiest ratio of macro-nutrients for good health and longevity is 30% fat, 15% lean protein, and the remaining 55% low-glycemic carbohydrates.

  As a general rule, any food scoring less than 55 is considered low GI. Dr. Allen's Glycemic Research Institute is the only FDA-approved GI certifier. The certification process tests foods for diabetic and nondiabetics, as indicated by these symbols. To date, hundreds of thousands of products have been tested for their GI, Dr. Allen says.

However, few companies are revealing their GI cards yet; most are waiting to see if the idea takes off as well as the Atkins low-carb craze.

Though there is but one official FDA-approved certifier, this hasn't stopped food manufacturers from touting their products as low GI, even without the FDA-approved testing. If you see products without the seal that claim to be low GI, there is no guarantee that the company's measuring tactics were valid or the tests did not favor product sales over health.

Proponents of the labels say that they are a valuable tool for managing weight and blood sugar levels. Critics cite inconsistencies with seemingly healthy foods like parsnips and watermelon, which have high GI values—since no one ever got fat eating parsnips or watermelon, the statistics leave room for false impressions if used improperly. The limitation of the glycemic index is that it doesn't take into account the amount of carbohydrates in a given food. For instance, per serving watermelon has a small amount of carbohydrates, but it ranks high on the GI scale. To counter this, researchers have developed the glycemic load, which takes into account the amount of carbohydrates in the food, thus reassigning foods like watermelon with an acceptable GI-load rating.

Although understanding just how the laboratory tests determine GI ranking is complicated, the general principles are not rocket science. It's the same advice our doctors and mothers have been telling us for years—eat plenty of fruits, vegetables, and whole grains and focus on healthy fats like those from fish and canola oil. It's not a very sexy message—which is why food marketers haven't promoted it to the extent of low carb, yet.

Bread and Cereal Labels

WHOLE GRAINS

If you have bad childhood memories of whole-wheat bread for its brick-heavy weight, bread science has overcome the downside of whole wheat. New brands with whole grains are remarkably light. This is achieved by adding dough conditioners, protein, new fibers, and yeast nutrients to hold up to the sturdy grains.

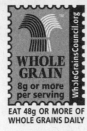

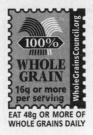

The Whole Grains Council and Oldways Preservation Trust, a consortium of mills, nutrition-minded chefs, and manufacturers, is working to improve the image of whole-grain breads and cereals with these trademarked black and gold stamps. The Whole Grain Council stamp states the number of whole-grain grams in a single serving for the product with a reminder that we should eat at least 48g of whole grains per day.

In addition to the fibers naturally found in plants, like wheat germ, bran, and psyllium, bread manufacturers are experimenting with fibrous filaments from the world of prebiotics. There is no easy definition of prebiotics, so stay with me here. Prebiotics are complex carbohydrates that pass undigested to the colon, where beneficial bacteria consume them and release vitamins, minerals, and nutrients—like I said, not easy to understand. Just remember that in this case, an additive called inulin is a positive attribute, since it acts like fiber and helps improve the immune system. Look for it in breads, cereals, and yogurt products.

In the cereal aisle, whole grains are everywhere. Even brands with the toys in the box have switched to whole grains; however, many of these are made "with whole grains." "With" is the key word here, for in some brands the fiber content is still a measly 1g.

For a truly valuable improvement in kids' cereals, look at brands that used to be sold exclusively in the health-food store. Now that many of these companies have been purchased by larger corporations the availability is better. For instance, General Mills purchased Cascadian Farms, Kellogg's bought Kashi; through Pepsi's acquisition of Quaker Oats they now own Mother's Natural.

Health-food purists see the trend as cashing out, but for consumers the mergers open up hundreds of new and healthier products to choose from on grocery store shelves. The products don't need a lot of detective work from consumers to see they are healthy. Particularly among the children's cereals, there are brands that are actually healthy *and* appeal to picky eaters—they even have fun characters on the box.

OAT CHOLESTEROL HEALTH CLAIM

In 1997, the FDA approved a health claim petitioned by Quaker Oats regarding the cholesterol-lowering properties of oats. The studies that supported the claim showed that eating 3g of beta-glucan per day in oats lowers blood cholesterol by as much as 5%. To get the full benefits you must eat what Quaker Oats calls a "good-sized bowl," or a serving and a half, of *whole* oats (¾ cup dry oats). That means whole oats, not processed oats.

This distinction hasn't stopped marketers from making claims. Here is one example:

Three grams of soluble fiber daily from whole grain oats foods, like Oatmeal Crisp Hearty Raisin, in a diet low in saturated fat and cholesterol may lower cholesterol and reduce the risk of heart disease. *Oatmeal Crisp Hearty Raisin has one gram per serving.*

OK, so they aren't lying, but plastered all over the box is "lower cholesterol." But you will have to read the fine print to see that one serving isn't enough to make your physician smile or your cholesterol go down. So if you eat instant oatmeal or most other processed cold oat cereals, you will need to eat three servings to get the recommended 3g of soluble fiber in whole oats.

The key to the oatmeal claim is soluble fiber. Fiber is divided into two categories, water soluble and insoluble. Insoluble fiber passes through the intestinal tract intact, hence its positive digestive properties. Soluble fiber is more bioactive, hence the recommendations to eat more. Soluble fiber binds with fatty acids and slows digestion so blood sugar is released more slowly. These binding properties help moderate LDL cholesterol by removing it from the body. Sources of soluble fiber include oatmeal, oat bran, barley, flaxseed, nuts, legumes, apples, pears, strawberries, blueberries, prunes, and citrus fruits.

REDUCED SUGAR

Walk down the cereal aisle of the grocery store and you're likely to witness an ugly scene—tantrums about too many tantalizing candy-coated cereals, and that's from the parents trying to fend off their children's begging pleas. In 2005, Kellogg's, Post, and General Mills introduced reduced-sugar versions of some of their most popular brands, like Fruity Pebbles, Cocoa Puffs, Trix, and Frosted Flakes. Parents were thrilled until they saw through the hype. The sugar had been replaced by other types of refined carbohydrates, like maltodextrin and dextrose, that were just as nutritionally void as sugar.

At present, ingredients like starches, which the body metabolizes like sugar, don't have to be listed in the nutrition panel as sugars. In the sugar shell game of labeling, manufacturers take away the high-fructose corn syrup (HFCS) or sugar and add in starches. However, the labeling laws allow these starches to be omitted from the sugar column on the food label—like I said, a shell game. So ignore the lower-sugar claims on the front; instead read the side panel.

The best advice I've seen thus far about cereals is from noted pediatricians and the authors of *Eat Healthy, Feel Great, The Family Nutrition Book,* and *Dr. Sears LEAN Kids,* Bill Sears, M.D., Martha Sears, R.N., and sons, Jim and Bob, also pediatricians:

1. Look for carbohydrate-sugar ratios of four to one. For instance, if the cereal has 24g of carbohydrates and 6g of sugar, it's a good buy.

2. Remember the five and five rule: 5g of sugar or less and at least 5g of fiber (dried-fruit cereals may have a higher sugar content than this and be OK—the labels make no distinction between added sugars and natural sugars in fruits).

3. Protein content should be at least 3g per serving.

4. Vitamin and mineral content, especially iron and zinc, should be 25 to 40% of the Recommended Daily Allowance (RDA).

HEART HEALTHY

The cereal aisle is full of brands with health claims for lowering cholesterol and keeping your heart healthy, while at the same time they contain hydrogenated fats (a manufactured fat that contributes to heart disease) and often too much sugar. The criteria to market products as heart healthy follow FDA-agreed-upon guidelines for "healthy," such as 3g fat or less, 1g saturated fat or less, 20mg cholesterol or less, 480mg of sodium or less, and at least 10% of the daily value (DV) for six nutrients (vitamin A, vitamins C, iron, calcium, protein, and dietary fiber).

In June 2006, the American Heart Association (AHA) released new diet and lifestyle recommendations; among the six new suggestions for a healthier lifestyle were to "reduce saturated and trans fatty acids in the diet" and "minimize the intake of food and beverages with added sugars."

With this recommendation in mind, it isn't clear why at the same time kid-appealing high-sugar brands of cereals, such as Cookie Crisp, Count Chocula, and Lucky Charms carry the AHA seal and are on its online shopping list. Or why brands such as Smart Start, marketed as part of the "Go Red for Women," are endorsed by the AHA when the ingredients include partially hydrogenated fats. (See the Addendum in the back for an update.)

There are many notable healthy cereal brands that carry the AHA symbol or are indeed heart-healthy cereals, like Fiber One, Cheerios, and Kashi—but since there are flaws in the criteria, read the ingredient panel for sugars and trans fats. Last, remember that manufacturers pay $7,500 and a yearly renewal fee to carry the AHA symbol, so remember that just because the label isn't present doesn't mean the brand isn't healthy—it simply may not be in the manufacturers' budget.

VITAMINS, LOW FAT, SUGAR-FREE . . .

Calcium, iron, vitamin C, thirteen vitamins and minerals, low fat . . . the list goes on. Cereal manufacturers can spray virtually any vitamin or mineral on the cereal they like, and most cereals are low fat anyway. These claims are fine, but they don't tell you anything about what's under the vitamins. Most often the more flashing signs on the box, the less nutritious the cereal. For instance, does it really matter if there is added calcium when the sugar content is sky high and the grains are refined?

Nutritionists tell me that there is still much confusion about carbohydrates, sugars, and calories, some of which came from the low-carb phenomenon. They advise consumers to look at sugar content, as well as total carbohydrates. The advent of new sugar substitutes means a product can easily be sugar free and filled with blood-sugar-altering carbohydrates. Most of all, they say, remember the DVs on the side of the box, especially for calories, are for a person who can consume 2,000 calories a day. Most women can live quite nicely on less, which means the calorie, carbohydrate, and fat percentages on the side of the box are not accurate for most females, so be conservative in your judgment.

Genetically Modified Grains

You may have read that GM foods have infiltrated our entire food supply. It's hard to know the actual numbers, since GM foods are not allowed to be labeled as such. With the lack of transparency in food labeling and the seemingly low-profile manner in which they were introduced into our food supply, one might assume that this notion is correct. The number that is bantered about most frequently is that 60 to 75% of all food products contain GM ingredients.

It's a matter of semantics—nearly all processed foods have some derivative of a GM crop. There are a dozen specific fruits and vegetables that have approval from the FDA to be sold as GM, though the two foods that dominate are corn and soybeans. This includes foods like corn chips, corn cereal, cornmeal, corn flour, and corn oil, as well as soybean oil and soy flour. Cornell researchers noted that if you add canola and cottonseed oil to that list, that brings the total to almost 100% of processed foods being made from a GM food.

Other plants such as rice, sugar beets, potatoes, zucchini, tomatoes, and papaya have patents for GM crops, however, with the exception of Hawaiian GM papaya, the crops are not widely planted because of consumer resistance or warnings from processors who say they can't export foods like sugar made from GM sugar beets. GM wheat may also be on the horizon, but farmers have been resistant to planting it because it reduces their ability to export to the E.U. and Japan, where GM grains are banned.

Genetic modification is perhaps one of the most contentious issues that pit the organic food industry against conventional farming. The complaints against the technology are many, including endangering wildlife, concerns about environmental and human safety, genetic drift, and superweeds.

There is a weed in my garden called bindweed that winds around every strawberry plant, corn stalk, and bean vine in its path. My belief, as a writer who covered the issue of genetic modification before the general public even knew what GM foods were, is that the heart of the controversy is that strong corporate interests, science, and politics are wound together tighter than the bindweed in my garden. Each strangles the other for fear that a hint of legitimacy might bloom from the controversy that favorably endorses one over the other.

Farmers choose biotech seeds for multiple reasons—including a belief they will prevent most crop-damaging diseases and provide higher yields and convenience. In 2004 as many as 85% of soy farmers planted biotech soy; this is a 73% jump from 1997. Some farmers are pleased with the convenience because the technology allows the application of weed killers without damaging the plant, although other farmers find the unforeseen consequences just as frustrating as unwanted weeds.

From an environmental perspective, GM crops may not be the ecological choirboy they were introduced as. One of the pro-GM arguments for crops such as corn, soy, and cotton was that it would reduce the amount of herbicides and pesticides used in farming. A Farm Bureau/Philip Morris poll of farmers and consumers in August 1999 indicated that 73% were willing to accept genetic engineering as a means of reducing chemical pesticides used in food production.

What the consumers in the study didn't realize was that for crops like corn and soy, the farmers are weighed down mostly with trying to control weeds, not insects—so pesticides are less an issue than herbicides. The newly developed GM seeds allow soy and corn farmers to apply glycophosphate herbicides, which kill weeds but not the plant. To their credit, glycophosphates do remain in the ground for less time than other more toxic herbicides. You are most likely familiar with the same home garden variety chemical, called Roundup.

So have GM seeds reduced chemicals, as farmers hoped and consumers desired? It depends on whom you ask. In the early years, from 1996 to 1998, GM crops reduced the amount of chemicals applied to crops by 25.4 million pounds. By 2004, this number exceeded 62 million pounds. However, in recent years, from 2001 to 2003, the amount of glycophosphate herbicides has climbed by 22%. The spike is because glycophosphate herbicides cost a lot less than they used to, so farmers can afford to spray more.

GM seeds have reduced the use of other more harmful insecticides for corn and cotton by as much as 19.6 million pounds. For cotton, used to make textiles and food-grade cottonseed oil, this change is important since the types of chemicals used are very toxic. The other plus is that GM crops require less tilling, so fuel emissions can be considerably less (Monsanto estimates that biotech farming has eliminated as much as 10 billion kg of carbon dioxide from the air worldwide). Organic agriculture has been criticized because of reliance on tilling, which can lead to erosion. But new machinery that crimps plants during harvest, rather than tilling, is proving a beneficial farming tool that doesn't disturb the soil. So again, the image of environmental savior is not altogether accurate.

Biologists have their own list of complaints. They contend that beneficial insects rely on many of the weeds that glycophosphates kill for survival and without them the eco-balance of biodiversity is disrupted. Another downside is that the overuse of the herbicide can create a superweed that is immune to chemicals—the concern is that it will take even more pounds of other, more toxic herbicides to keep weeds under control.

"Weeds have a way of fighting back," says my dad, Jim Archer. He also says that the only initial advantage that he sees is that GM seeds allow for easy weed control, but every year the disadvantages add up to higher unforeseen costs. GM seeds cost more per acre to plant and they cannot be replanted from year to year, as farmers fear steep fines from the seed company. In addition, farmers pay technical fees—for every bag of GM seed farmers buy they pay an additional ten to twelve dollars to the seed company. Farmers in foreign countries don't pay the same technical fees, he says, which means imported soybeans can be less expensive than U.S.-grown beans. In addition, the promise of higher yields for GM crops hasn't always held true—the differences in some crops are minute.

For farmers who choose to grow non-GM seed the biggest obstacle is a problem scientists call gene flow, where GM traits drift or creep to non-GM crops from wind and insect pollination, sometimes traveling as far away as twelve miles. To date, the litmus test for whether GM crops can coexist with organic crops (by law organic certification prohibits GM farming)—and even non-GM crops grown by conventional farmers—hasn't been positive because there is virtually no way to prevent the phenomenon. Tactics like buffer zones are mandatory, but it's impossible to prevent wind, bees, birds, and insects that spread the modified genes from trespassing.

Non-GM and organic farmers bank on the higher prices they receive for their crops; however, on more than one occasion farmers didn't find out that their non-GM grain had been infiltrated by biotech genes until they tried to sell it, only to realize their crop had been downgraded to lesser commodity prices. More and more farmers who sell to export markets, like rice to Japan and wheat to Europe, say the risk is too great to allow widespread use of GM crops.

If you add it all up, higher prices for seeds, fines for replanting seeds, technical fees that go to the seed company, more toxic herbicides to control superweeds, limited export markets, and lower commodity prices for GM crops, simply for the convenience of spraying glycophosphates, may not be worth it. My father used to grow Roundup Ready Soy, but he is so disgruntled with it all that he has let his 100 acres go fallow for the first time in the farm's 100-year history. In his mind, the only real winners are the GM-seed and chemical companies.

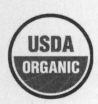 From a consumer perspective, the biggest fault of GM technology is a lack of transparency. Too many questions were left unanswered before the technology was so freely introduced. Ultimately the FDA says it is up to the food producer to prove that a food is safe for consumers and the environment, a contention that has been violently protested by non-GM activists.

Had the science of genetic modification been introduced in a more well-designed and transparent manner than how it happened perhaps the reception would have been less hostile. A succession of botched experiments such as adding Brazil nut proteins to soybeans and recalls of toxic GM potatoes pressed consumers to ask: Who is in charge? Tree nuts are among the top five allergens in this country, and potatoes are well-known for their toxic properties without adequate controls.

Allergic reactions remain a top concern because the newly designed food may unwittingly introduce a new allergen to a consumer. GM supporters say this possibility is virtually nil because of extensive testing. The biotechnology industry claims they are developing technology to rid problematic foods of allergens altogether. Since there is no foolproof way to predict food allergies without individually testing each person for every new GM food, the debate will likely continue.

When introduced, the science of genetic modification was primarily interested in the process of adding genes to plants, rather than the safety of the newly designed food. Authors Nina Federoff and Nancy Marie Brown outline the most commonly held beliefs and myths about GM technology in their book, *Mendel in the Kitchen: A Scientist's View of Genetically Modified Foods*. They explain that at the time the technology was launched to the public there was a big disconnect between the fields of plant science and nutrition. The assumption, they say, is that since all allergens are proteins, every transferred protein used in GM foods must be first considered an allergen.

This hasn't always been the preferred protocol, nor has careful oversight prevailed. A big blunder allowed GM corn for animal feed, called StarLink corn, to infiltrate the human food supply, which resulted in massive food recalls of corn products. Allergic reactions were reported, although the CDC could not confirm the validity of the claims.

Four years *after* StarLink, in March 2005, the journal *Nature* reported that for years a strain of genetically modified corn that did not have regulatory approval for human consumption had also entered the food supply. This time, the corn strain, called Bt10, was inadvertently allowed into the human food supply for as many as four years. The slip equaled only about .01% of all the corn planted in the United States during that time, and the specific strain did not pose any risk to humans. The company Syngenta discovered the mistake and reported it immediately to the EPA and USDA. However, since there was no health risk, both agencies decided to not report the incident to the public. Again consumers ask: Who is in charge?

The FDA's failure to allow labeling of "GMO-free" foods has been heavily criticized, as genetic modification is considered a "right to know" issue. Their inaction smacks of a double standard, since terms like "fat-free" are allowable but not "GMO-free," and irradiated foods must be labeled with the radura symbol, so why not label GM foods? The inconsistencies have pegged the FDA with a reputation as a puppet of the biotechnology trade. For the consumer, the current situation leaves few choices. If you prefer to avoid GM grains, the only way to do so is to buy certified organic products and products that are labeled with "We do not use ingredients that were produced using biotechnology."

GRAINS CHART

Men mastered the science of farming as far back as the Stone Age, when they grew enough grains to get them through the winter. Some of these ancient grains are back in food fashion, notably for their protein and adaptability for just about any cuisine. Whole grains are known for their ability to reduce heart disease and regulate the digestive system— somewhere in the low-carb craze we forgot about their healthy properties and culinary versatility. Here are a few you've probably seen on store shelves and wondered what they were and how to use them.

The Nitty-gritty on Whole Grains		
What	Why	How
Amaranth	Peppery flavor, complete protein, gluten free.	Muffins, pancakes, wheat breads
Barley	Lowers cholesterol as well as, or better than, oats.	Salads, stews, chili, side dishes
Buckwheat	Although this is a fruit related to the rhubarb, it's treated like a grain. Has high levels of an antioxidant called rutin, which improves circulation and removes unhealthy cholesterol.	Pilafs, breads, baked goods

What	Why	How
Bulgur	Wheat kernels, usually durum, that are boiled, dried, and cracked. High in fiber. Polished bulgur is called *grano*.	Hot cereal, meatless burgers, salads, puddings
Corn	High levels of antioxidants; corn treated with alkali in hominy and masa harina (used to make tortillas) is high in niacin. Look for whole-grain varieties instead of degerminated, which is not whole grain.	Popcorn, tortillas, corn bread, stews
Farro (Emmer)	Ancient wheat eaten by the Roman legions. Soak overnight for best results.	Soups, mixed with greens and cheese, side dish
Kamut	Nicknamed King Tut's wheat because of its ancient origins. Buttery tasting, high in protein and vitamin E.	Use flour like wheat in breads, desserts, and pasta. Toast before cooking.
Millet	Most often seen in bird feeders—try it anyway. It cooks up well when mixed with other grains.	Add to other grains in breads and stuffings. Toast before cooking and don't overcook.
Oats	To retain the wholeness of oats, buy steel-cut and thick-cut rolled oats. Rich in cholesterol-reducing beta-glucan and an antioxidant that protects against unhealthy cholesterol.	Cooked cereal, add to cookies, bars, breads, pancake batter, meat loaf, meatballs
Quinoa	Cultivated by the Incas, now grows in Colorado. A botanical relative of Swiss chard. Perfect	Rinse, rinse, rinse before cooking to remove a soapy-tasting coating.

(continued)

What	Why	How
	protein that contains all the amino acids the body can't produce on its own.	Use in Southwestern side dishes with chiles, corn, and tomatoes.
Rice	Easily digested, gluten free. Look for black, purple, and red rice varieties. Whole-grain rice retains all the fiber and vitamins; converted rice (parboiled rice) has more B vitamins than regular white rice.	Whole-grain rice in pilafs, limitless uses . . .
Rye	High fiber, low GI.	Rye flour in bread; prepare rye bulgur similarly to wheat.
Wild Rice	Seed of an aquatic grass, native to the Great Lakes area. Twice the protein and fiber of brown rice.	Use with other types of rice; allow for 45 minutes' cooking time.

Bottom Line

My boys' favorite daily errand in the Italian village where we once lived was to visit the baker. They ran faster than I could keep up down our cobblestone-paved hill to Franco's bakery. By the time I caught up, they were perched on flour sacks, nibbling on cookies and singing Italian nursery rhymes. For me, the biggest readjustment when we returned stateside was the bread and pasta—no more racing down the hill, no more local pasta or freshly baked bread, and no more singing with Franco. The fervor that vilified the two foods was implausible. I am fairly certain that if Franco were our national baker, no such myth would exist.

Bread's bad reputation for its ability to impale our bloodstream with excessive sugars was from our never-ending attempt to process food into its barest components; this time the highly processed, spongy white breads were the laboratory equivalent of pure white sugar. I'm hoping for a little more clarity, cool heads, and a hands-off approach to our food in this new millennium. So far, the ever-increasing availability of whole-grain breads is impressive.

Ever since I was old enough to fight with my little brother for the free prize, I've been a cereal box reader . . . Bullwinkle comics on the backs of Cheerios and who can forget the twenty-five-cent tugboat offer on the Rice Krispies box? I've replaced my breakfast reading companions of Bullwinkle the moose and Rocky the squirrel with the morning newspaper, yet cereal boxes are still great billboards: "can help lower cholesterol," "12 vitamins and minerals," "may reduce risk of heart disease," "good source of protein," and "whole grain." The selection, the advertising, and the claims are a credit to the doggedness of the American advertising industry. Just like in the bread department, there are some healthy whole-grain cereals shoehorned in among lights, bells, and whistles. If nothing else, follow the Drs. Sears' advice, five for five—5g of sugar (or less) and 5g of fiber (or more)—ignore the moose and squirrel.

CHAPTER 8

Change Your Oil

Inroads to Good Health

"Take the Via Appia and turn left at the Cleopatra Bridge," I told my husband. At the turn, recollections from the once-familiar road jolted our memory. Journalists have at least one story in their career that leads them to unexpected places and people. For me it was olive oil.

On this fall day, the path had come full circle. Years before I became a journalist, as a U.S. Navy wife stationed in Gaeta, Italy, I traveled this section of the Old Rome Road daily, to take my kids to soccer practice or to explore the coastline along the Tyrrhenian Sea. As in the biblical days when Peter and Paul walked the road in their sandaled feet, the Via Appia is still the best vantage point from which to anoint oneself in local culture.

The Americans stationed in the area named the decrepit bridge that marks the turnoff to the autostrada the Cleopatra Bridge. Our romantic notion was that Cleopatra crossed the river here while living in one of Caesar's villas outside Rome—doubtful but a good story.

As many good stories do, my adventure back to Cleopatra's Bridge started with a rumor. The gossip among food writers was that the reputation of perhaps the noblest fruit of all, the olive, was bruised by corruption and greed. My hope was that olive oil maker Antonio Marulli and Catherine Amey, an Italian-American couple living only minutes from my former Italian home, would lead me to answers, or at least rumor control.

After a long lunch, Antonio and Catherine drove us to the family's olive estate. Narrow roads cut between fields of tall corn and low-lying swamps that are home to water buffalo, prized for *mozzarella di bufala*. As we entered the estate, volcanic dust, the decimator of Pompei, powdered the car with sienna red soil. The Campagna province is known for growing sugar-sweet tomatoes, dazzling blood oranges, and impressive olives. Antonio's trees were no exception, as the green fruit hung heavy on the branches.

I was there because of Antonio's allegiance to creating high-quality extra-virgin olive oil (EVOO) in a region known for mass production. Neighboring farmers grow only a few olive varieties; Antonio grows seven different species. The variation gives his oil a distinct flavor— fruity with a subtle spiciness. "When I first started," Antonio says, "my neighbors didn't think something this serious could be done. But now they see many people from France and England coming here to buy my oil."

During October and November, he and his staff handpick the olives just before they ripen. In the evening, mini Fiat pickup trucks deliver the green pearls to a friend's mill—the only one Antonio trusts. He insists on a state-of-the art centrifuge mill. Stone mills are for tourists, not high-quality EVOO.

After pressing, the oil is scrutinized by members of an expert tasting panel who verify that it meets flavor and aroma standards set by an Italian association of small-estate oil producers. Olive oil experts say that blending and fermenting skills make man the master of wine, but the flavor of EVOO is reliant on a higher power, solely at the mercy of the soil, the weather, and the olives. Only after Antonio's oil passes the panelists' tests can it carry the estate's Monte della Torre label; then he can breathe a little easier.

Antonio fills a bottle with *olio novello*, the season's first pressing. We taste it by the spoonful and dip chunks of bread into the streams of green oil. It tastes bright and slightly pungent—markers of a fresh and healthy EVOO.

I ask Antonio if the rumors are true. He chooses his words as carefully as his olives: "Let me put it this way: It's impossible to buy a good-quality extra-virgin olive oil in a plastic bottle for three dollars."

He explains that it costs a certain bottom-line figure to make EVOO, from any country, so be wary of prices that are too low.

Caveat Emptor

From here, this nugget of suspicion led me back to Italy three more times. Each visit revealing a complex yin and yang industry—one side is marked by small estates such as Monte della Torre; the other side is a complex infrastructure of tankers from Tunisia, Morocco, Turkey, Spain, and Greece delivering oil to Italy.

Italy's reputation as the world's largest supplier of olive oil isn't entirely true. Spain holds that title. Since growers can't make enough EVOO for even their own citizens, Italian olive oil companies rely on other countries, largely Spain, to meet the world's demand. Italy is more like the central spigot for olive oil.

Companies with Italian-sounding names, such as Bertolli and Berio, funnel imported oils with a fraction of genuine Italian EVOO into bottles and stamp them with the label "Imported from Italy." While there is nothing inherently wrong with this practice, don't be misled into thinking that these oils are 100% Italian and paying more than you should.

It wasn't until a New York lawyer, Marvin Frank, filed a class action suit against the olive oil giant Bertolli that the label "Imported from Italy" got some clarification. Frank charged that deceptive labeling and marketing misled consumers into thinking the olives were grown, pressed, and bottled in the Italian motherland.

In 2001, Frank offered an olive branch, agreeing to settle the case, provided Bertolli oil tagged as "Imported from Italy" also list the oil's countries of origin—Spain, Greece, Tunisia, and Turkey. The case prompted other suppliers to do the same.

E.U. and Italian agricultural officials say the thousands of fraud cases per year cost the government millions of euros. Deceptive labeling is minor; more costly ruses include suppliers' blending EVOO with other oils to stretch profits. Unless blatant, it's difficult to trace adulteration. A supplier can get away with adding as much as 5% hazelnut oil to EVOO because the chemical structures are so similar that it slips by testers' microscopes. Add a drop of canola oil to olive oil and the scam is over.

Another technique is to add old or low-quality olive oils to EVOO. Only recently has science caught up with the adulterers. Through optical fingerprinting, the same technique doctors use to measure oxygen in your blood, the industry can finally answer the age-old question of virginity, at least for olive oil.

Domestic Disturbances

Stand in front of the olive oil section in any grocery store and you are likely to see oils from small estates rubbing labels with large multinational products and private label brands. The price and quality differences are vast and competition is fierce.

Grocery and specialty store retailers bear the brunt of the good and bad decision making along olive oil's long chain of custody. For instance, a gourmet store owner, requesting anonymity, told me a scenario that may be all too common. While looking for Italian oil to sell as a store brand, the retailer made inquiries to a U.S. bottler with a warehouse full of Turkish oil. When the store owner declined his wares because the oil wasn't Italian, the bottler pointed to the drums of Turkish oil and replied, "I can label this Italian, no problem."

Private label brands can be more about price than quality. Suppliers of EVOO say that demands for lower prices, especially for private label brands, open the doors for unethical practices. At times the wholesale prices, decided on by supermarket contract negotiators, are set below production costs (about six dollars a liter), meaning the only way to win the bid is to sell lower-quality oil as EVOO. Just as Antonio warned, you can't buy good-quality EVOO for three dollars a liter, or even six dollars.

As California's olive oil industry moves from boutique business to nationwide distribution, the California Olive Oil Council (COOC) reports similar problems. Although on a much smaller scale, unprincipled bottlers label imported oil as Californian. "Some believe that in order to survive in this industry, you have to check your morals at the door," said Jamie Johansson, owner of Lodestar Farms, an olive oil maker in Oroville, California. "It's like selling California peaches and saying they're from Colorado," he said.

In response to the problem, the COOC has adopted ethics rules for its members and is holding dodgy suppliers accountable with lawsuits. In addition, the group pushed the USDA to update U.S. olive oil standards and labeling rules, which hadn't been changed since the 1940s. Until the USDA standards are approved, little will prevent importers from sending us low-grade oil and successfully passing it off as extra-virgin to naïve American consumers.

Change Your Oil, Often

When Italian villagers need olive oil, they fill jugs directly from the vats at the olive orchard. The oil is as fresh as a flirtatious shoe salesman at the village open-air market. Here in the States, the quest is not nearly as fun. The fine print is our only guarantee of freshness and quality, and knowing just how to interpret the text can mean a difference in your health.

To grasp the health properties, think of the oil as simply the juice of the olive, like orange juice. Oil pressed from old or damaged olives contains fewer active ingredients, such as antioxidants and polyphenols, known to improve longevity and health. Lower cancer rates, healthy hearts, and strong joints are only a few of the reasons you should use EVOO.

If you're asking, "How long has it been since I used that extra-virgin oil in my cupboard?" it may be time to invest in a few new bottles. Within one year most of the healthy components decrease sharply, and within two years rancidity is likely. As with wine, there are high- and low-end oils, each one with its own culinary purpose, so you may need to buy more than one bottle. In my cupboard, you'll find high-quality oils for drizzling on salads or cooked vegetables, an everyday EVOO for sautéing, and a light-flavored virgin oil for baking.

P-A-G-E-D

The easiest way to read EVOO labels is to remember the acronym **PAGED: Price, Acidity, Geography, Extra-virgin, and Date.**

Price   A reasonable cash outlay for good-quality EVOO is fifteen to twenty-five dollars a liter. Reserve these oils for adding to fresh salads, finishing cooked vegetables, sprinkling on grilled meats and fish, and light sautéing. Blended oils from many countries cost about eight dollars per liter and are useful for cooking recipes such as spaghetti sauces and stews.

Acidity   The International Olive Oil Council (IOOC) in Madrid mandates that EVOO must have an acidity level no higher than .8%. Suppliers are beginning to list acidity on the labels.

Geography   In general, EVOO made from a single country or region and approved by an agricultural agency is higher in quality than oils blended from various countries. For perfectly fine everyday oils, look for oils from single countries. For fine-quality finishing oils to use on salads or vegetables, look for oils from single regions such as Tuscany or a locale in Spain or Greece. They will all say "Product of . . ." "Italy," "Spain," or "Greece," for example. Each country likes to say they produce the best—all are very good—so as with wine, find a few brands you like.

Extra-virgin   Extra-virgin olive oils are made from olives grown and pressed using very specific guidelines for harvesting and pressing— the more careful the process, the healthier the oil. Pure olive oil is highly refined and shouldn't be confused with EVOO.

Date   By the time some oil reaches U.S. shelves it could already be a year old; then after it sits in a warehouse rancidity isn't far off. After twelve months even unopened EVOO loses a significant portion of its health benefits. Try to find the most recent date possible, either a sell-by date or a Julian calendar bottling date. If a date isn't visible, ask your retailer; the backroom paperwork may reveal the oil's birthday.

Scusi? Are You a Virgin . . . Label?
Olive Oil Labels

Since there is a vast difference in the quality of EVOO, a trend in third-party labeling has begun. The labels are designed to give you some assurance that the oil is made using guidelines that meet or exceed international standards.

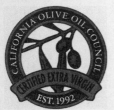

CALIFORNIA OLIVE OIL COUNCIL
This olive oil label is monitored by the COOC, an association of olive growers and oil suppliers. The group has no tolerance for olive oil adulteration and deceptive labeling. Its members must comply with ethical principles and are held accountable if they fail to meet the standards. COOC-labeled oil exceeds the parameters set by the IOOC for acidity and flavor.

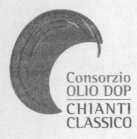

CHIANTI CLASSICO BLACK ROOSTER
Oils produced in the Chianti Classico region of Tuscany have high standards of quality, as seen on the black rooster wine labels. Not just hype, the standards set by the Consorzio del Marchio Storico-Chianti Classico for EVOO exceed those of the IOOC for quality, flavor, geographic denomination, and environmentally friendly growing methods.

APPELLATION D'ORIGINE CONTRÔLLÉE (AOC), DENOMINACIÓN DE ORIGEN PROTEGIDA (DOP), DENOMINAZIONE DI ORIGINE PROTETTA (DOP), HELLENIZ FOREIGN TRADE BOARD (HEPO)
These French, Spanish, Italian, and Greek appellations denote that the olives were grown and the oils pressed in well-defined geographic regions with specific growing methods. Each geographic label is overseen and verified by an association of E.U. agricultural officials, growers, and olive oil experts. The labels are similar to appellation labels used for wine.

USDA ORGANIC CERTIFIED

Organic EVOO, domestic or imported, carries a seal from a USDA-accredited organic inspection agency, such as Quality Assurance International (QAI). It may also have a USDA organic seal, but this is voluntary. Organic European bottled EVOO will have an Agriculture Biologique (AB) logo, a guarantee that E.U. organic rules were followed; the rules are similar to USDA organic standards.

In cooler climates, olive trees don't need many, if any, pesticides; however, trees in warmer climates are prone to olive flies, which require chemical or natural pesticides. Some farmers don't use pesticides but choose not to certify their orchards as organic because of the expense. If you see the words "made with organic olive oil" without a seal or certifying agency, 75 to 95% of the oil is organic.

OLIVE OIL HEALTH CLAIM

The FDA approved a qualified heart-health claim in 2005 for pure olive oil:

> Limited and not conclusive scientific evidence suggests that eating about 2 tablespoons (23 grams) of olive oil daily may reduce the risk of coronary heart disease due to the monounsaturated fat in olive oil. To achieve this possible benefit, olive oil is to replace a similar amount of saturated fat and not increase the total number of calories you eat in a day.

Pure olive oil is one of the healthier refined oils because of its high monounsaturated fat content, known to reduce cholesterol levels. However, it should not be confused with EVOO, an even healthier oil that contains monounsaturates, as well as polyphenols, antioxidants, and healthy fatty acids.

Pure olive oil is made by refining the pulpy remnants (skin, pits, and olive flesh) of EVOO. The refined oil is called crude pomace, a tasteless oil used to lubricate machinery. The oil isn't fit for human consumption until some EVOO is added back in.

You may like the milder taste of pure olive oil, but it's that kick in the back of your throat from EVOO that means the oil is alive and healthy. In my opinion, the health label is a disappointment because it makes no distinction between extra-virgin and pure olive oil. While pure olive oil is healthy liquid fat, the healthiest benefits are stripped away during the refining process. It's a little like using the same coffee grinds over and over. Eventually there is nothing left that resembles its original contents except tinted water.

OLIVE OIL Q & A

What is "cold pressed"? "Cold pressed" is a marketing term that has little meaning. It used to refer to the temperature restrictions during extraction from stone mills or hydraulic presses. Today most EVOO oil is coaxed from the olives using computerized centrifuge mills with controlled temperatures.

Does light olive oil have fewer calories? "Light" olive oil has just as many calories as other olive oils. "Light" refers to the mild taste due to the small amount of EVOO added back into the oil after refining.

How should I store olive oil? First, look for oil in dark green bottles and metal cans; they protect the oil from the 24/7 supermarket lights, which can cause degradation. Once at home, store the oil away from heat in a dark place (a metal oil can will keep the temperature down, if stored in the dark). If you refrigerate EVOO, the cold temperatures will slow down oxidation and preserve the polyphenols longer; it will not, however, prevent rancidity within the oil's two-year life span. Refrigeration congeals the oil; it will take about an hour to bring the oil back to room temperature.

Is unfiltered oil better? Filtration is a matter of preference, not a measure of quality. Unfiltered oils have bits of the olive fruit floating in the oil, which can alter the taste.

Does color matter? Don't judge an EVOO by its color. Depending on the soil, the climate, and the olives, the color will vary from an iridescent green to a golden yellow.

Should extra-virgin olive oil taste peppery? Yes. Depending on where the olives are grown, the oil leaves a spicy note in the back of your throat, which is a good thing. In general, oils made in areas with cooler climates, such as Tuscany, have a peppery flavor; those made in areas with milder climates have a softer flavor. If your oil smells moldy, like Play-Doh, it's most likely rancid.

Can I fry with extra-virgin olive oil? EVOO has a lower smoke point than seed oils, so it's best to use virgin oil for pan frying and refined olive oil for high heat. All fats undergo chemical changes under high heat, although olive oil, in all its forms, is more resistant to these unhealthy changes than some seed oils. An oil chemist told me he fries with a blend of three-quarters pure olive oil and one-quarter EVOO, because his own kitchen laboratory tests show that the healthy components in EVOO transfer to the food. There aren't any large studies proving this, but it's an interesting idea.

No Longer the "F" Word—Healthy Fats and Oils

As you can tell, EVOO is on the top of my shopping list when my kitchen oil can is empty. Perhaps my Greek heritage and love for Italy make me biased. However, I do buy other types of cooking oils. When I crave blueberry muffins on a Sunday morning or Kung Pao on a Friday night, olive oil just won't do.

The first lesson in culinary oils is to let go of all of your preconceived notions about fats. Forget low fat and no fat; instead get your mind around words like "mono," "poly," and "essential fatty acids." The skinny on fat is that liquid fats, those found in the baking aisle of your supermarket, play an important role in good health.

We all need fat to survive. Without it our blood pressure and heart rate would go awry, our blood wouldn't clot, and our nervous system would forget to fire off impulses that keep us going. Fats also keep our hair and nails healthy, protect our organs, and move fat-soluble vitamins A, D, E, and K from food into our cells. That aside, fatty foods taste good and make us feel satisfied.

There are four types of fats—saturated, monounsaturated, polyunsaturated, and trans fats (hydrogenated)—each listed on the labels of culinary oils. Fats are defined by the type of fatty acids that hold the chains of fat molecules together, each one with an explicit task. For instance, first-rate fatty acids maintain levels of HDLs, which protect the heart by sweeping away damaging LDLs that stick to artery walls. Deadlier fats favor LDL production and should be eaten sparingly.

Unfortunately, oil labels don't tell you which fats to avoid and which you should get to know. Even so, the scientific language of fats isn't conducive to eye-catching marketing messages. Fats are definitely easier to eat than understand; this primer will shed some light on how to read an oil bottle from back to front.

Changing Your Oil for Life's Mileage

The goal for overall good health is to limit intake of saturated fats to no higher than 7 to 10% of your total calories. If you ignore Julia Child's advice and stave off butter whenever possible, you may think you don't eat saturated fats, but even liquid vegetable oils contain some saturated fats. Oils with the lowest saturated-fat levels include a patented oil called Enova (.5g/tblsp), high-oleic safflower and sunflower oil (.8g/tblsp), and canola oil (1g/tblsp).

Next in line are avocado, sunflower, corn, extra-virgin olive, refined olive, grape seed, and macadamia nut oils (1.3–2g/tblsp). Nut oils, such as hazelnut, walnut, almond, and pumpkin seed, are also low in saturated fats. Refined nut oils are stable enough for cooking; unrefined nut oils break down, so reserve these for dressings and adding to already-cooked foods.

TRANS FATS

My great-grandmother taught my mother to make pies with lard. Somewhere down the span of generations, probably during the low-fat craze, we switched to vegetable shortening. Like a Mary Poppins piecrust promise, "easily made, easily broken," we should have listened to the wisdom of time-honored traditions.

It turns out that when seemingly healthy vegetable oils are turned into vegetable shortening (or partially hydrogenated oils) by adding a hydrogen molecule, the transformation doubles our chances of developing heart disease, insulin resistance, and diabetes. Partially hydrogenated vegetable shortening contains a whopping 18% trans fats, while lard has only 1%. In addition, the naturally occurring trans fats in lard, and even butter, may be less deadly than laboratory-made shortening.

If you can't stand the thought of using lard, coconut and palm fruit oils are good alternatives to vegetable shortening. After decades of using tropical fats, scientists saw that saturated fats from coconut and palm fruit did not raise unhealthy cholesterol levels. It's important to buy palm fruit oil, rather than palm kernel oil, which has almost double the saturated fat. If you are still loyal to vegetable shortening, Crisco recently introduced a trans-free product, made from vegetable oils and fully hydrogenated cottonseed oil. Foods made with fully hydrogenated fats are cholesterol neutral—meaning they will not raise bad cholesterol or lower good cholesterol.

Be aware that the latest FDA rulings for trans fats allow manufacturers to say their products are "trans-fat-free, per serving," if there is less than .5g per serving. If the oil contains, say, .45g of trans fats, it qualifies for the clause. If you consistently eat more than the recommended serving, you may be eating more hydrogenated fats than you realize. In June of 2006, FDA announced they may drop the limit of allowable trans fats to .2g. Comments are under review; if approved, manufacturers will have to reformulate their products (once again) if they want to make the "trans-fat-free, per serving" rule.

MONOUNSATURATED FATS (MUFAS)

Monounsaturated fats lower LDL cholesterol levels without negatively interfering with helpful HDL levels. The abundance of monounsaturated fats is the primary reason the Mediterranean diet is one of the heart-healthiest choices possible.

Although the label won't tell you, the type of MUFA that is the most beneficial is omega-9 fatty acids. This fatty acid helps EVOO fight off cancers, balance healthy cholesterol levels, and support immune function. Omega-9s are in high-oleic safflower, sunflower and canola, extra-virgin olive, avocado, nut, and sesame oils.

POLYUNSATURATED FATS (PUFAS)

Polyunsaturated fats are the reason we cannot entirely eliminate fats from our diet. These fats are necessary for life and are only available through food, which is why they are called essential fats. Embrace these fats in moderation. Physicians now know that without these fats our arteries harden, our blood pressure skyrockets, and we run out of energy, but too much isn't good, either.

That said, it's not enough to look for only polyunsaturated fat contents on the label, because PUFAs are further broken down into unique fatty acids, some we should get more of, others less. The most abundant PUFA is linoleic acid, also called omega-6 fatty acids. Although we need this fat, most likely we get way too much of it through processed foods. To counter the imbalance, physicians recommend that we eat more fats that contain omega-3 fatty acids (such as ALA).

For optimum health, we *need* a 1-to-1 ratio of omega-3 to omega-6 fats; we *get*, on average, a ratio of 1 to 20, because of all the processed foods that use fats with omega-6 fatty acids. Canola, avocado, nut, flaxseed, and hemp oils contain notable levels of omega-3s to right the proportion.

Big Fat Labels

Reading fat labels seems a lot like a high school chemistry class. If you stick with it, getting comfortable with the vocabulary can be well worth it for your long-term health. In addition to poly, mono, and saturated, here are other labels to get to know.

Diacyglycerol Oil This newly introduced oil is a blend of canola and soy oil, manipulated so that our body absorbs less fat. Sold as the patented Enova brand, the oil is high in the fatty acid diacyglycerol (DAG) and low in triacyglycerols (TAGs), a fat our bodies use rather efficiently. For most cooking oils the opposite is true. Studies on Enova show that the DAGs slide through the intestinal tract unnoticed; the remaining 20% of TAGs are absorbed. The oil is still as caloric as other oils, so use sparingly. Don't confuse this with Olestra, an oil used in snack food production, with molecules so large that none ever get absorbed in the intestine (see more in chapter 12).

Expeller-Pressed A majority of seed oils are extracted using high-heat phosphoric acids and hexane (similar to dry-cleaning fluid), which evaporate during the extraction process. Expeller-pressed oils are hydraulically extracted using a chemical-free process and refined with low heat and citric acid (vitamin C). Tests show that expeller-processed soybean oil is just as stable as highly refined oils with added preservatives, making it a good choice for frying and repeated use.

Genetically Engineered Canola If you browse the Internet for information about canola oil, no doubt you'll find a host of Web sites spouting the dangers of canola oil. The overblown conspiracy theory reiterates a myth that canola was created through genetic engineering and is poisonous.

Canola's tainted reputation is based on junk science stirred with a hefty dose of old wives' tales. In truth, genetic engineering, where genes are inserted from a different plant into a host cell, is a relatively new technology. Canola is more than thirty years old and was created using old-fashioned hybridization, the same science you learned in sixth-grade science class. A 3,000-year-old plant, rapeseed, was selected for its desired traits and cross-bred with other plants, resulting in seed that produces a healthy, low-fat oil.

This is not to say that there isn't genetically engineered canola; just more than half of all canola is now genetically engineered to tolerate the herbicide Roundup, as is a large percentage of corn (40%), soy (81%), and cottonseed oils (71%). The FDA does not require manufacturers to label ingredients as genetically modified. If you prefer to avoid GE cooking oils, look for organic certification, which forbids the use of GM seeds.

As for poisonous? . . . Impossible. Many of the rumors claim that canola rapeseed is toxic—more rubbish. Most seed oils have alternative commercial uses depending on how they are processed. For instance, flaxseeds are the foundation for linseed oil or a very healthy dietary supplement; corn oil has hundreds of uses, including ethanol and cooking oil; even crude olive oil is used for machine lubrication and for pure olive oil. Canola is derived from a nontoxic species of rapeseed. If all rapeseed species were toxic, you couldn't eat kale, rutabagas, or turnips, which come from the same family.

High Heat   Oils have different smoke points, literally meaning the maximum temperatures before the oils begin to smolder. However, no oil should be heated past its smoking point because then the chemical structure begins to degrade and the oils release carcinogenic free radicals. Some fats have a naturally high smoke point, peanut oil for instance; others are refined to increase the smoke point and are labeled as high-heat oils.

High Oleic   High-oleic oils are made to produce oils that are higher in monounsaturated fats and lower in saturated and polyunsaturated fats, making them more heart healthy than their parent plant counterparts. High-oleic oils include canola, safflower, and sunflower.

No Preservatives   Some oils have added preservatives such as BHT, BHA, and TBHQ to extend shelf life. While these ingredients are approved by the FDA, there is concern about their safety and many consumers prefer to avoid them. Studies are ongoing to find more "natural" ingredients to replace them. Brands sold as expeller pressed do not contain preservatives.

In a nutshell, you want to buy oils that are low in saturated fats, high in monounsaturated fats, high in omega-9s and omega-3s, and low in omega-6 fatty acids. With this in mind, here are the oils that meet the criteria.

Oils	Low Saturated Fats	Monounsaturated	High Omega-9	High Omega-3	Low Omega-6	Purpose
Canola	X	X	X*	X	X	All-purpose
Macadamia Nut	X	X	X	X	X	All-purpose
High-Oleic Safflower and Sunflower	X	X	X		X	All-purpose
Olive	X	X			X	All-purpose
EVOO	X	X	X		X	Avoid high heat
Enova†	X	X				All-purpose
Grapeseed	X	X	X			All-purpose
Avocado and Nut	X	X	X	X	X	Refined OK for high heat
Flaxseed and Hempseed	X	X	X	X	X	Not for cooking

* Spectrum Naturals sells canola oil with high omega-9 and low omega-6 levels.
† Patented canola and soy oil that reduces fat absorption.

RECIPE FOR CHANGE

By substituting liquid oils for butter and margarine you can reduce your saturated fat intake by more than half and overall fat intake by 25%. For baking, use lighter-flavored oils in cakes, muffins, and pizza dough; cookies need a blend of liquid and hard fats for best results.

Butter or Margarine	Liquid Oils
1 teaspoon	¾ teaspoon
1 tablespoon	2¼ teaspoons
¼ cup	3 tablespoons
½ cup	¼ cup + 2 tablespoons
1 cup	¾ cup

Source: Canola Association, www.canolainfo.com.

FUNCTIONAL OILS

Flaxseed oil was at one time reserved only for dietary supplement use. Flaxseed oil is rich in ALAs (omega-3s), known to help soothe joint pain, calm the raging symptoms of menopause, and regulate blood lipid levels.

Manufacturers recognized that it takes a significant number of pills to get the maximum benefits and now sell the oil in bottles. A tablespoon of flaxseed oil may be good for your health but tough to swallow. For a more palatable option, blend it into salad dressings. By adding a few tablespoons to a good EVOO, wine vinegar, a bit of mustard, fresh herbs, and seasonings, you'll increase the health properties significantly, and no one is the wiser, except you.

You can find bottled flaxseed oil in the refrigerated section in the supermarket, usually near the yogurt. Flaxseed oil goes bad quickly, so look for a sell-by date distant enough to finish off the bottle within a six-month window.

Some flaxseed oils claim to be high in lignans, the fibrous outer shells of the flaxseed, which are high in antioxidants and components useful to fight annoying menopause symptoms, like hot flashes. Manufacturers add lignans back into the oil because they are stripped away during pressing, but if lignans are important to you, it's best to use ground flaxseed.

CHAPTER 9

Baker's Dozen

Is the Honey Industry a Sticky Mess?

The whole life process of ants and bees is fixed down to the smallest detail by rigid, hereditary instincts, the social pattern and interrelationships of human beings are very variable and susceptible to change.
EINSTEIN, *MONTHLY REVIEW*, NEW YORK, MAY 1949

This story started out as sweetness and light on a summer afternoon, until a conversation on a beekeeper's back porch revealed gray clouds in an industry that deserves better. No matter how much you remember about the magic of bees and honey making, the honey world is not all sweetness and light, as it should be. It's about predators, price dumping, and honey laundering.

I met Tom Theobald, a Boulder, Colorado, beekeeper and president of the local beekeeping association, in his backyard, an iced tea in one hand and a camera in the other—between us sat a transistor radio with the battery panel open. I couldn't resist asking. . . . "Just wait," he said. Beekeeping is a job of patience; journalism isn't—I waited eagerly nonetheless.

A few minutes into our conversation, Theobald's guest of honor arrived, putting it all into perspective. A bee hummed inches over our heads, with bits of soft white fluff in her clutch, and flew straight for the radio. Theobald snapped a few shots of the winged creature as she slipped into her new home. Using the same flight pattern, she returned every ten minutes to fill her single family colony with downy treasures. It was pure magic and a fitting end to the sweet side of the story. "It's not about the honey," Theobald said. "That's the bonus. It's about pollination."

Pollination, the mystifying instinctual vocation of bees, has been threatened by years of pesticide exposure, parasites, destruction of habitat, invading Africanized bees, and economic incentives to buy cheaper imported honey. Theobald is used to losing a small percentage of hives every year to natural causes. But when the numbers climbed to 30%, qualms arose that neighboring farmers were spraying pesticides without warning beekeepers, as they should.

Theobald is known for his stinging opinions about our state's beekeeping industry. His arguments and official filings with state agricultural workers about pesticides are often played out in Colorado newspapers, but officials say it's difficult to pin anything on farmers unless they are caught in the act. Since by nature honeybees visit flowers across several square miles it's often impossible to pin down the exact location of the problem. Nevertheless, once the damage has been done, the only thing to show for it is dead bees—a situation that constantly frustrates Theobald.

Overall, about 20% of the nation's bees have been lost to some degree of pesticide and insecticide exposure. As bees gather nectar, the pesticides cling to the bees' outer coat, spreading to other bees when they return to the hive. Bees don't reproduce quickly enough to recover from insecticide exposure, since it can take as long as three years. Adding to the injury, for years bees have been plagued by a blood-sucking mite that killed off as much as half of the North American bee population. Research is honing in on a solution, but again it will take years for beekeepers to recover from the damage.

As more bees disappeared from the rural landscape, orchard farmers who once relied on native bees, nature's free pollination service, turned to renting hives. The situation became so dire that California and Northwestern tree farmers looked as far away as Florida and Australia for healthy bees to pollinate their crops. Since as much as one-third of the American diet is reliant on pollinators, Canadian botanist Dr. Jim Kemp likens the value of bees in orchard farming to "a $20 bill flying by." It's more like $20 billion flying by; that's the economic impact of bee pollination for crops including almonds, apples, melons, plums, blueberries, cherries, pears, cucumbers, cranberries, and kiwis, as well as dairy and meat, since alfalfa and clover need bees as well.

The demand for pollination has transformed beekeepers' staid routines of packing honey to a nomadic lifestyle of chasing the seasons. In the middle of Colorado's winter, Lyle Johnston, beekeeper, melon farmer, and former president of the American Honey Producers Association, loads his bee colonies onto trucks and heads west until he reaches the San Joaquin Valley in California for almond pollination season. As soon as the bees' work is complete, Johnston packs them up again and heads north to Oregon and Washington for apple, pear, cherry, and berry season, finally returning to Colorado for melon and honey packing season.

It's Not About the Honey

It's not enough that mites, pesticides, and sprawl put bees at risk for endangerment—our own foreign trade policies really sting beekeepers. Until 1995, imported honey from Argentina and China was tightly controlled to about one-third of overall volume by trade agreements. During the latter half of the decade two problems converged—American bee colonies and native bee populations began to die off, and there was little interest on Capital Hill in renewing trade agreements to cap honey imports and continue domestic price guarantees. Honey importers and commercial food makers took advantage of the policy changes, especially since China's and Argentina's honey making production costs were 30 cents per pound lower than those of American beekeepers. The sharp rise in cheap imports forced American beekeepers to give up. American beekeepers no longer came close to producing enough honey for their own country's consumption, which also meant a decline in pollination for crops that need bees.

Down but not out, the American Honey Producers Association, led by Johnston at the time, organized a campaign to save domestic honey from demise. Their efforts were rewarded when, in 2001, the

International Trade Commission (ITC) ruled that international honey imports threatened the livelihood of the remaining 2,759 American beekeepers. The ITC imposed tariffs on honey from Argentina and China, upping imported honey prices by as much as 184%, a closer match to U.S. production costs. The decision pitted domestic honey suppliers against importers who were happy with the cheaper prices and healthy profit margins.

A series of sticky events following the ITC tariffs further soured honey imports. Customs inspectors discovered Chinese bulk honey imports were contaminated with low levels of chloramphenicol (CAP), a potentially harmful antibiotic and nonapproved food additive. The investigation also uncovered a circuitous route Chinese exporters were using, shipping honey through Asia and Australia, to bypass the importation tariffs.

If this weren't enough, Chinese honey exporters needed a profitable way to get rid of the CAP-contaminated honey. They did so by filtering out the contaminants, leaving a sticky syrup called ultrafiltered honey. Once again, the ultrafiltered honey was shipped through intermittent seaports before arriving at U.S. docks. Officials were tipped off when countries began exporting more honey than they produced, by as much as 4 million pounds per month. To add suspicion, countries like Singapore, with no known commercial bee population, became substantial honey exporters almost overnight.

Laboratory tests further sealed the case when in 2004 13% of sixty-nine samples of imported honey were identified as an altered product rather than real honey (seven from China, one from Turkey, one unknown). No one is certain how much ultrafiltered honey was sold as pure honey; most officials suspect it was sold to commercial food makers for breads and cereals.

Perhaps the country most hurt by the price-dumping charge was Argentina, where beekeeping is a jumble of cottage industries and larger exporters, with little government support. South American critics of the U.S. move cried protectionism, citing that Argentina's beekeeping industry is too poor and fragmented to come up with such an organized plan of price dumping.

Unfortunately, Argentina's beekeepers were caught in the middle of a Chinese government-supported beekeeping industry and an alarming decline of the American bee population. At the risk of over-simplifying, the move *was* protectionism—it protected the American farming system. If this were simply about honey prices, it would be fair to argue about unfair trade practices. If there aren't enough bees, our food supply for fruits and nuts may be as dependent on foreign imports as we are for oil. It's not about the honey; that's the bonus. It's about pollination.

Made in the U.S.A.

Now that the honey industry has dealt with declining bee popula-tions, tariffs, and honey fraud, one might hope that they are getting back to the days of full barrels. Not so fast; there is still the issue of la-beling. If I asked you to define "honey," the reasonable answer would be something like "the golden, sticky substance taken from a bee-hive," right?

The definition depends on whom you ask. The word "honey" sells, so food processors label a product as containing honey even if there is no or little honey in the product. Products like honey crystals, honey syrup, and, my favorite sham, sugar-free honey are just a few honey imposters on the shelf.

Surveys show that when a product label uses the word "honey," consumers prefer it over other brands. Shoppers may see the word "HONEY" in big letters on the front label, but the back panel lists corn syrup well before honey. There's no telling how much honey is in the product, if any at all—think of honey-glazed ham, honey cough drops, honey mustard salad dressings, honey barbecue sauce, and honey-sweetened cereals. If honey is listed at the tail end of the in-gredients, there is a good chance only a fraction of honey is present.

Sellers of the real stuff say honey labeling should be all or nothing. But there is little regulatory control or USDA support. For instance, when the last USDA honey chemist retired in 1978 the position re-mained vacant. If there are any government rules, they are less strin-gent than the honey industry would like. For instance, FDA guidelines suggest that if honey is the characteristic flavoring, honey should be 10% by weight—but the ruling isn't closely enforced.

If you want to support American beekeepers and our entire tree and crop farming system, buy U.S.A.-labeled honey and local honey. Honey packers aren't required to tell you where their honey comes from, but most U.S. companies display their origins proudly. If there is no country of origin, even if the packer is from this country, assume all or some of it is from overseas. Also be aware, if the honey is imported and the price is extremely cheap, it may not be honey at all.

Sugar and Flour Labels

Ever since we were tall enough to reach the cookie jar and old enough to have our first cavity filled, our relationship with sugar has been bittersweet. Scientists recently discovered a gene that triggers the tongue to recognize sweet treats, so it seems that we are hardwired to love sugar. A gene to justify our cravings is good news, but it doesn't offer a glimmer of hope that eating as much sugar as we want to might be good for us.

Unfortunately, the next few paragraphs aren't going to tell you that, either. Alas, sugar should be eaten in moderation. Still, there are a fair number of rumors and labeling ticklers milling about that might make us think that one type of sugar is better for us than another. As much as they might try to convince you, granulated sugar is still sugar. On those occasions when only a sweet will do, here is what you need to know to find just the right sugar to satisfy a sweet tooth and your baking needs.

SUGAR

Sugar comes from cane or sugar beets, and both need a fair amount of refining to extract the sugar from the plant's fibers. Niche market brands would like you to think their sugar is not processed; it's not true. Their processes are different, but sugar of all types is refined. Sugar is just too dirty to eat in its raw state.

Cane sugar goes through two processes. The first takes place at the cane fields, where raw sugar is extracted from the fiber. At a mill, raw sugar is heated and treated with phosphoric acid (the same flavoring in colas) and lime (the calcium hydroxide used in corn tortillas) to separate out the impurities. At this point the sugar grains are yellow.

Here is where myth and reality meet. Bone char (electrically charged pieces of burned cattle bones) is used to filter and whiten the crystals. This practice is particularly offensive to vegetarians, even though all traces of the bone are separated out. Today most cane sugar refineries have switched to a granular activated charcoal, the same type in home water filters, aquariums, and water treatment facilities. You'll have to call the specific sugar manufacturer to find out if they use bone char or charcoal. If it's any consolation, the bone char process is approved by kosher certifiers since it's completely removed from the sugar.

If bone char is still something you prefer to avoid, beet sugar is not subjected to bone char, ever. It's made by washing and cutting sugar beets into shoestring potato slices, heating the juice, and separating the impurities from the sugar with lime. Beet sugar is whitened with diatomaceous earth (a sedimentary rock).

Evaporated Cane Sugar   Evaporated cane sugar is a favorite choice for natural-food lovers. Often the term "raw sugar" is used to describe these brands. True raw sugar isn't safe for human use, so this is simply a marketing term to get your attention. Other types of evaporative cane juice sugars include Demerara and Turbinado—the tan color varies by the amount of molasses coating the crystals.

Evaporated cane sugar undergoes a refining process that uses evaporative methods to separate the sugar crystals from the debris. Sugar made from this process retains some molasses, trace minerals, and B vitamins, but it is hardly a good source of nutrients. This sector of the sugar industry is known for environmentally friendly growing methods: certifying the sugar as organic and committing to regenerating the cane waste for electrical power and cane field fertilizers.

Brown sugar   Brown sugar is made by retaining some of the molasses in the cane sugar; "light" and "dark" refer to the amount of molasses. Brown sugar from beet sugar is refined sugar with molasses painted on the crystals. Muscovado is the truest of brown sugars because the molasses is embedded in the sugar crystals; it has a strong molasses flavor and fine crystal grain.

Cane and beet sugar can be used interchangeably in most cases. My father, who farms sugar beets, will hate to read this, but professional bakers say cane sugar is better suited for sugar syrups, the caramelized crust on crème brûlée, angel food cakes, and some sponge cakes. The chemical structure of beet and cane sugar is almost exactly the same, but the last little .05% may yield different results depending on the recipe. Manufacturers aren't required to say whether the sugar is beet or cane. Unless the package is labeled as cane sugar, there is little way to know. Even within the same brand, the company may switch sources depending on price and availability.

ALTERNATIVE SWEETENERS

The range of alternative sweeteners, other than sugar, honey, and maple syrup, is a constantly expanding sector of food science. You will need some time to experiment when baking to find out how these compare to granulated sugar—a one-for-one substitution is not the best advice; start with one-quarter or one-half and go from there.

AMASAKE is fermented sweet brown rice syrup, good for puddings, smoothies, and sweet sauces. Baking will take some kitchen detective work.

BARLEY MALT OR BROWN RICE MALT SYRUP is made from sprouted barley or rice. Good for baked beans and puddings. Leavened baked goods need experimentation or a good cookbook.

DATE SUGAR is granulated sugar made from ground dates. It does not dissolve well in liquids, so it's best in heavier recipes, such as quick breads and muffins, and sprinkling on top of pies and fruit desserts.

FRUCTOSE is made from fruit sugar or corn syrup. There is a widespread debate about how the fruit-derived and corn fructose affects blood sugar levels. Fruit-derived fructose is half as sweet as sugar (half sucrose, half glucose), leading some to think it's a healthier choice than cane or beet sugar. Although it's structurally different, physicians warn that since it is still a concentrated sweetener, so you should eat it as sparingly as granulated sugar (see the soft drink chapter for more on high-fructose corn syrup). Substitute half a cup of fructose for every cup of sugar, suitable for all purposes.

FRUITSOURCE is the brand name for a sweetener made from grape juice concentrate and rice syrup. It's a fat replacer as well as an alternative sweetener. Use cup for cup with sugar, reduce fat by half, and keep oven temperatures between 300 and 325 degrees Fahrenheit.

HONEY varietals include clover, eucalyptus, fireweed, orange blossom, sage, and tupelo. It is sold as pasteurized (heated to prevent yeast growth) or raw (nonheated). Neither form should be fed to children under the age of one because of a risk of infant botulism. Substitute half to three-quarters of a cup of honey for each cup of sugar, add one-eighth teaspoon baking soda, and reduce liquid by one-quarter cup.

MAPLE SYRUP is tapped and boiled sap of sugar maple trees. Syrups are graded by the USDA as follows: Grade A Light Amber (fancy grade) is light and mild, an early-season syrup; Grade A Medium Amber is a bit darker, with more maple flavor, often table syrup; Grade A Dark Amber is darker and stronger still, a late-season syrup; Grade B (Cooking Syrup) is very dark, with a strong maple and caramel flavor, and holds up well in baking and cooking. Substitute three-quarters of a cup for one cup of sugar; add one-eighth teaspoon baking soda.

MOLASSES is derived from cane sugar and is notably the most nutritious sweetener of all because of calcium, iron, B_6, and potassium. The three types are based on the age of the sugar cane and the order of extraction: unsulphured is made from the juice of ripe cane and is extracted during the first pressing; sulphured comes from less mature green cane and is treated with sulphur fumes during extraction; and last, blackstrap is extracted from the last boiling phase of the cane; it is known for a strong flavor and high iron content. Substitute one and a half cups unsulphured and sulphured molasses or slightly less blackstrap for each cup sugar. Increase baking soda by half a teaspoon.

STEVIA is derived from the leaves of a South American shrub and estimated to be 300 times sweeter than sugar. Stevia cannot be sold as a sweetener in the United States because of FDA concerns about its safety. With SWAT-style actions, the FDA has tried to shut down stevia manufacturers, but the product continues to be sold in stores as a dietary supplement. The sweetener is noncaloric, and as little as one teaspoon of powder or liquid can be substituted for each cup sugar (one-quarter teaspoon stevia for one tablespoon sugar).

SUCANAT is an evaporated cane sugar with molasses. Works well in cookies and bars, but it doesn't dissolve completely, making it tricky for light cakes and leavened breads. Substitute one for one with sugar.

ARTIFICIAL SWEETENERS

A lot of chemistry happens when ingredients like flour, sugar, and butter get together, which is why baking with artificial sweeteners is tricky. Each of these products can replace sugar, but you may lose some of the recipe's original integrity. For instance, cakes need a balance of sugar and fat for a nice crumb, so go easy and leave time for mistakes (to read about the safety of these ingredients, see the beverage chapter). For best results, substitute any one of these products for no more than half the sugar.

Ingredient	Tolerates Heat	Amount
Acesulfame-K	yes	12 packets for ½ cup sugar
NutraSweet	no	Substitute one for one; packets are more concentrated than pourable product
Saccharin	yes	8 teaspoons for 1 cup sugar
Sucralose (Splenda)	yes	½ cup for each cup sugar

FLOUR

All-purpose flour   This is the workhorse of bakers' kitchens. However, not all brands are exactly alike; switching brands may yield different baking results because of protein. Most national brands have about 11 to 12% protein. Midwestern and Northern brands are generally higher in protein, while Southern and Northwestern brands are as low as 7.5 to 9.5% protein.

A labeling requirement allows flour manufacturers to round up or down to the nearest gram for protein—the small difference is enough to make a recipe flop. For example, actual protein content may be 2.7g (per ¼ cup), but the label says 3g. Similarly, the protein may be 3.3g (per ¼ cup) but the label says 3g. It seems like a trivial complaint, but the differences can add up. For instance, the 2.7g protein flour adds up to 10.8g for a full cup (which is considered low protein) and the 3.3g protein totals 13.2g per cup (which is considered high protein). But both of these brands will say 3g protein on the label.

This 2.4g disparity defines the difference between an all-purpose flour and high-protein flour. You may think you're having a bad baking day, but it might be that you chose a different brand of flour. The best advice is to stick with a brand if you like how it behaves—or vice versa. Check the protein content in your flour if your recipe flops.

Bleached or Unbleached?   Professional bakers prefer flour with some aging behind it because young flour makes for weak gluten. The process takes a few weeks to occur naturally, and while this happens the flour tends to yellow. Mills use chlorine gas to speed up the aging process and peroxide to whiten the flour. Unbleached flour doesn't undergo this chemical process, which is why the flour has a yellow hue.

Bromate   Bromate is added to flour and baked goods to strengthen dough. Under improper conditions, such as using too much and not cooking the bread long enough, bromate can cause illness. The Center for Science in the Public Interest has asked for a ban on bromate in flour because it is a suspected carcinogen. The FDA has asked flour companies and bakeries to voluntarily remove the ingredient from products. Look for flour that is labeled as "never bromated" or "non-bromated," as well as baked goods *without* potassium bromate or bromated flour. Most companies now use ascorbic acid for the same results, but bromate is still used (in 2003 children in nine different schools in Massachusetts became ill after eating flour tortillas made with bromated flour).

Pastry Flour   Pastry flour is low protein (8–9%) and is usually unbleached. Whole-wheat pastry flour can be substituted for half of the white pastry flour with good results.

Cake Flour   Cake flour is a soft, low-protein flour (7–8%), perfect for light cakes with a tender crumb. Most cake flour is bleached because the chlorine gas toughens the protein, which helps the flour literally hold up more than its weight in fat and sugar. As a substitute for cake flour, remove two tablespoons of all-purpose flour from each cup and replace it with cornstarch. Bleached all-purpose flour is also a close substitute, but the cake's texture will be a bit heavier.

Bread Flour   Bread flour gives yeasted breads a strong skeletal structure to hold their shape during rising, baking, and cutting. Hard winter red wheat contains 12–13% protein, which creates enough gluten to produce a light and airy loaf. Some brands contain ascorbic acid (vitamin C) to improve the rise.

Whole-Wheat Flour   Whole-wheat flour contains wheat germ, bran, and endosperm that are normally stripped away in white flour. The germ contains the bulk of the vitamins, protein, minerals, and polyunsaturated fats, and the bran is rich in fiber. Newly developed white whole-wheat flour is light in color and texture but nutritionally equal to harder wheat varieties. The biggest downfall of whole-wheat flour is that it doesn't rise as well as white. To overcome this, add a few tablespoons of vital wheat gluten or a commercial bread enhancer, made from gluten, vitamin C, and malt (available from specialty stores).

Stone-Ground Whole-Wheat Flour   Stone-ground whole-wheat flour is reminiscent of our grandparents' day, when local wheat was milled down by the river under a stone grist mill. The advantage is that more of the vitamins and minerals in the germ are preserved. If you want truly stone-ground wheat look for 100%, because some mills blend stone-ground with machine-milled wheat and call it stone-ground.

Self-Rising Flour   Self-rising flour contains baking powder and salt, suitable for quick breads, pancakes, and biscuits. Bakers report mixed results with self-rising flours because there is no way to know if the leavening power in the baking powder has lost some of its strength. To make your own, add one and a half teaspoons baking powder and a half teaspoon salt for every cup of all-purpose flour.

Instant Flour   Instant flour is made by precooking the flour's starch molecules and drying it again. The process makes for an easy-to-use thickener that can be added to hot liquids and sauces at the last minute. The flour also works well as pastry board flour when rolling out dough; the granules keep the dough separated from the rolling pin and the surface.

Semolina   Semolina isn't a type of wheat; it's the endosperm of durum wheat (the hard wheat used to make pasta). It is high in fiber and protein and thus produces strong gluten bonds for hearty, chewy bread. The flour is available in fine or course ground.

Spelt Flour   Spelt is an ancient European grain, gaining popularity in the United States, especially among people with sensitivities to traditional wheat. Although the grain is still technically wheat, some people find it more agreeable to their digestive system than traditional hard red wheat. Spelt flour's protein levels are as high as 17%, making it a good replacement for whole wheat.

Gluten-Free Flours   Gluten-free flours are useful for people with celiac discase, which causes an inability to digest gluten, resulting in mild to severe digestive and malnutrition problems. To make gluten-free breads and desserts requires a cupboard full of creative leavening ingredients including xanthan gum, guar gum, and methylcellulose, which give the bread elasticity and stability. Without these additives, you can replace only about 20% of the regular flour with gluten-free flour. Look for specialty cookbooks to explain all the details. Gluten-free flours include corn, oat, potato, rice, and soy.

Chocolate

If there ever was a good food news story, it's that chocolate is actually good for you. Our low-fat obsessions and love-hate relationship with sugar obscure the fact that under all that angst is a healthy, antioxidant-rich food. There is a list of good things that chocolate can do for us, improving blood vessel linings and arterial stiffness, neutralizing free radicals (the unstable molecules that can damage cells and DNA), reducing hypertension, calming coughs as well as codeine, and, last, lessening diarrhea. Not bad for a food that every American woman had been told to avoid since puberty. There is a catch: It has to be either very dark chocolate or pure cocoa. Cacao pods are put through a vicious cycle of smashing, fermenting, drying, roasting, and grinding to remove the pod and pulp from the bean. While this goes on, much of what makes cocoa good for us is destroyed.

This health news was enough to make chocolate makers look at their manufacturing methods more closely and make some changes. There are plans to introduce a better grade, thus healthier, chocolate, in the near future. In the meantime use real cocoa for baking and beverages and eat the darkest chocolate you can find (70% cocoa or above).

DUTCHED OR NATURAL COCOA?

The process from cacao pods to cocoa powder involves roasting and grinding the cacao beans and pressing out the cocoa butter. This process leaves an acidic cocoa powder that can taste bitter, which is where dutching comes in (named after a Dutch chocolate maker).

Dutched cocoa is treated with an alkaline, which reduces the bitterness. Natural cocoas are known for stronger flavors and imparting a dark, rich color to baked goods.

The difference between dutched and natural cocoa is important in leavened baking, since some recipes rely on the natural acids in natural cocoa to react with the baking soda. Dutched (alkalized) cocoa might not create enough of a reaction and the recipe may taste soapy and bitter. If the recipe calls for natural and you have dutched cocoa, add a bit of baking soda to the recipe to precipitate a reaction. If the recipe doesn't specify, either type will do.

UNSWEETENED, BITTERSWEET, SEMISWEET, OR MILK?

Technically the American food grade system makes no distinction between bittersweet and semisweet. Both must contain at least 35% chocolate liquor. Most are closer to half; some are as high as 70%. Despite the lack of regulation, chocolate types within the same brand will reserve the name bittersweet for brands that have the higher amounts of chocolate liquor.

Milk chocolate has the most sugar and the least chocolate liquor and is softened with milk solids or condensed milk. White chocolate isn't chocolate at all, since it doesn't contain any cocoa. It's a mixture of cocoa butter, milk solids, and sugar. White chips often contain palm oil in addition to or instead of cocoa butter, which technically disqualifies them as "white chocolate," which is why you won't see the word "chocolate" on the label.

Bottom Line

It's difficult to imagine how the failure of one single product in the grocery store could bear the weight of the entire food chain—but our new national motto to protect the U.S. farming system should be "Save the Honeybee." This one tiny being holds up the entire U.S. farming economy, plants, poultry, and hoofed animals. There are a few simple changes you can make in your daily life to help make this happen: First, buy U.S.-made honey, preferably from local beekeepers; second, be cautious about the pesticides that you apply to your garden. Bees don't have boundaries; they might make a pit stop at your yard on the way to an orchard or farmer's field. These highly sensitive insects take whatever you put on your garden back to the hive.

CHAPTER 10

Towers of Babble: Canned, Boxed, Bagged, and Frozen

Climbing the Tower

For years food journalists complained that the food pyramid wasn't doing much for the American diet. Subjects like obesity, hypertension, and heart disease competed for disease-of-the-week stories in print and on television. So when the buzz began that a new food pyramid was about to be released, we were hoping for something that would set the fat-, salt-, and sugar-laden food industries on end.

Perhaps it wasn't as big as *Vanity Fair's* announcement of Deep Throat's identity. Food journalism isn't nearly as exciting as Woodward and Bernstein's realm; but as I waited for the news to show up in my computer in-box, I did wonder, would the USDA scrap the pyramid altogether and go for a new-age symbol of, say, macrobiotics and yoga (the symbol formerly known as the pyramid)? Or perhaps a new shape, one that reminded us less of our increasingly expanding pyramid-shaped bodies?

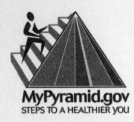

Instead we got another pyramid, this one color coded and being conquered by a lithe stick figure climbing what looks like the USDA version of Machu Picchu. The food pictures were gone, and for the first time the pyramid offered good advice for physical activity, real portion sizes, and an emphasis on high fiber, healthy fats, low-fat dairy, and lean proteins.

You might not have noticed it, but beans got two headlines—in the green triangle under "vegetables" and the purple sliver to the far right in the meat category. Also, hidden deep within the fine print of the dietary guidelines was a message to eat three cups of beans per week. Imagine, the humble bean, the wallflower of the canned food aisle, grabbing the spotlight from the more popular golden kernel canned corn or its younger cousin, the green bean.

The positive message was fortuitous for the Beans for Health Alliance, a public health, research, and public relations vehicle for bean growers and manufacturers. The same week the new food pyramid was released, the alliance gained approval from the FDA for a dietary guidance message that touted the benefits of eating beans to reduce the risk of heart disease and certain cancers. Now it's on the labels of canned and dried beans as well as canned, boxed, and frozen meals and soups that contain at least 50% beans.

A dietary guidance message is a broad dispatch designed to help consumers make healthy choices. It's a lot like advice from your mother—it must be truthful and not misleading, like "eat your vegetables," but without the motherly look and the finger wagging. "The great thing about this type of message is that it is simple and clean, and validates choices that healthy consumers are likely to make anyway," says Stacey Zawel, Ph.D., executive director of the Beans for Health Alliance. To date there are two approved messages of this type, one for fresh, frozen, and canned fruits and vegetables and the second for beans—both are attached to lower risks for cancer and heart disease.

The bean dietary guidance message was relatively easy for the Bean Alliance to obtain. There is little argument that beans are healthy and we should eat more of them, never mind the social drawbacks. Approval for other types of health claims remains difficult. They give the food world indigestion because their impact matches the complexity and economic implications of trade agreements with the E.U. The FDA files are packed with documents from food associations, politicians, consumer watchdog groups, and everyday people regarding proposed and approved health claims—each with their own passionate plea for approval or denial.

Nutrition Facts

Serving Size 1 cup (228g)
Servings Per Container 2

Amount Per Serving	
Calories 260	Calories from Fat 120

	% Daily Value*
Total Fat 13g	**20%**
Saturated Fat 5g	**25%**
Trans Fat 2g	
Cholesterol 30mg	**10%**
Sodium 660mg	**28%**
Total Carbohydrate 31g	**10%**
Dietary Fiber 0g	**0%**
Sugars 5g	
Protein 5g	

Vitamin A 4%	•	Vitamin C 2%
Calcium 15%	•	Iron 4%

* Percent Daily Values are based on a 2,000 calorie diet.
Your Daily Values may be higher or lower depending on
your calorie needs:

	Calories:	2,000	2,500
Total Fat	Less than	65g	80g
Sat Fat	Less than	20g	25g
Cholesterol	Less than	300mg	300mg
Sodium	Less than	2,400mg	2,400mg
Total Carbohydrate		300g	375g
Dietary Fiber		25g	30g
Calories per gram:			
Fat 9 • Carbohydrate 4 • Protein 4			

So begins the journey through the inner sanctum of the grocery store. On the back, side, and front panel of practically every can, bag, box, and frozen item are labels that have been designed by the wisest minds in nutrition, influenced by the craftiest minds in marketing, and monitored by empirically minded officials at FDA.

The Birth of Nutrition Facts and Health Claims

You may not remember it, but prior to 1990 that handy little nutrition panel describing calories and nutrients was found on only about one-third of foods. Even so, more than 40% of all foods had some sort of health claim—true or otherwise. In 1990, Louis W. Sullivan, secretary of health and human services, described the situation as "A Tower of Babel," requiring consumers to have degrees in linguistics, food science, and mind reading to understand the founded and unfounded claims.

While even now it may seem useful to have a modern-day Aristotle handy when deciphering food claims, it's less like Babel than it used to be. About 98% of all foods have the nutrition facts panel, and the number of health claims is better managed since Congress approved the Nutrition Labeling and Education Act (NLEA) of 1990. The NLEA sought to bring lawful order to food labeling by bringing consistency to how the nutrient content panel is displayed, defining terms like "reduced fat," and allowing for health claims, as long as there was significant scientific agreement (nutrient content claims will be discussed later in this chapter).

Since then, many of the health claims found on packaged and fresh foods came out of court cases and legislation from an unlikely source—the vitamin and supplement industry. The original NLEA document requested health claims for foods like fruits and vegetables and four dietary supplements (calcium, zinc, antioxidants, and omega-3 fatty acids). Of the supplements, only calcium was approved; the rest were shot down for lack of "significant scientific agreement." The denial set the tone for a movement led by dietary supplement manufacturers to classify supplements as foods, rather than drugs—a change the FDA never dreamed would happen.

Eat More . . . Vitamins?

For decades the FDA tried to twist the vise tight and regulate supplements as drugs, but they were up against a formidable foe. Dietary supplement companies were founded by a generation of entrepreneurs who learned the power of persuasion from civil rights and Vietnam War protests. They applied the same passion to their products and lobbied Capitol Hill and consumer groups by campaigning that Americans might lose their right to purchase dietary supplements because of the FDA's desire to regulate them as drugs. The crusade was energized by proposed legislation called the Dietary Supplement Health and Education Act (DSHEA) and was fueled by hundreds of thousands of public comments, which were, at the time, the largest lawmaking response ever recorded.

Whether supplements would have ended up solely behind the pharmacist's counter is debatable, but Congress bought the argument, every last little bit, largely because of the support from Sen. Orrin Hatch (R-UT) and Congressman Bill Richardson (D-NM). The passage of DSHEA removed any immediate hope the FDA had of regulating dietary supplements as drugs, judging them instead as food—just liked canned peas, with a few new rules.

The DSHEA victory led to a series of unpredictable events that no doubt kept FDA officials awake at night. It certainly kept me busy. I began my food journalism career during this health claim revolution. One of my rookie jobs was to write copy for food and dietary supplement products for a health-food trade publication. In addition to a Webster's dictionary and an Associated Press style manual, a dog-eared photocopy of DSHEA was never far from my desk.

For hours a day I pored over marketing and advertising copy and perfected a new vocabulary, born from DSHEA, called structure/ function claims, such as "may help reduce headaches" or "eases digestive trouble." Such claims were allowed as long as they didn't imply treatment or curative powers for diseases.

The biggest loophole was that structure/function claims didn't have to meet established guidelines outlined in the NLEA. Take frozen carrot cake for instance. When Kellogg's released a new line of pastas, frozen entrées, and desserts made with oat bran, called the Ensemble line (now defunct), the carrot cake carried a structure/ function claim stating it was "made with a natural soluble fiber that actively works to promote heart health," never mind that the other ingredients contained too much fat to make a substantiated heart disease claim.

It seemed that with each new claim I interpreted, a new court case emerged challenging the FDA's interpretation of the new rules of order. For instance, is pregnancy or menopause a disease? And should a supplement be sold as a food, even though it contains an active ingredient very similar to a drug? In the end, the courts sided with supplement manufacturers, allowing for structure/function claims under most circumstances, as long as they did not imply diagnosis, cure, or treatment of a disease.

While this was going on, the Food and Drug Administration Modernization Act of 1997 (FDAMA) passed, authorizing nutrient content claims, such as "low-fat" or "a good source of fiber," as well as health claims for conventional foods, provided they were substantiated by a U.S. government body or the National Academy of Science. Now, for instance, manufacturers may claim that orange juice, which is naturally high in potassium, may reduce the risk of high blood pressure per a thumbs-up statement from the National Academy of Science.

The cascade of fresh claims inspired new product developers. Now that supplements were food, why not sell food as supplements? Food companies interpreted the ruling as a go-ahead to supersede approval processes for ingredients Generally Recognized As Safe (GRAS) and began marketing food as supplements. Press releases came across my desk for chicken soup with echinacea, "to support the immune system," candy bars with ginkgo biloba for "enhanced energy," and even corn chips with kava; what was I supposed to say about these—"for relaxed snacking"? No amount of protesting, free-speech letter writing, or Capitol Hill lobbying could convince me that medicinal herbs in my soup or junk food were a good idea, even if the label said so.

Then DSHEA took a direction few predicted. Early pioneers of the dietary supplement and health-food industry, who supported DSHEA, had a utopian vision for the American consumer—dietary supplements and healthy foods that countered the status quo of conventional medicine and processed food manufacturing. But while supporters reveled in the passage of DSHEA, they didn't see that the light at the end of the tunnel wasn't a train at all—it was a computer monitor.

An entirely new type of entrepreneur came from a parallel universe called the Internet—a virtual store that didn't need approval from a suspicious store owner, grocery buyer, or editor bound to the rules of DSHEA. Better yet, their labeling, marketing, and advertising copy traveled under the radar screen of the FDA and Federal Trade Commission (FTC). For these manufacturers, structure/function claims were better than a preapproved line of credit. Almost overnight miraculous products sprang up on Web sites, preying on vulnerable groups looking for cures for chronic illnesses and quick weight loss from "breakthrough" supplements and foods.

Today the elaborate claims are more contained, largely due to surfing sweeps from the FDA and the FTC—and, I hope, smarter consumers. Most food companies have wisely given up selling food as dietary supplements with the exception of some meal replacement bars, beverages, and herbal infusions (teas). The core players in the health-food industry set such high standards for dietary supplements and food production long before the general public knew of the dangers of foods like trans fats and high-fructose corn syrup, and antibiotics in meat production—it's a shame that their mission was derailed with snake-oil tactics.

Healthland Security Advisory System—Threat Level, High

The most recent claim, a qualified health claim, is a declaration that appears to be true, but the evidence isn't 100% conclusive. It's hard to believe that the FDA would ever allow such a thing. When qualified health claims were approved, then–FDA commissioner Mark B. Mc-Clellan, M.D., strongly believed that claims met by a "weight of scientific evidence" were as useful to public health as the more stringent requirement for "significant scientific agreement," thus encouraging the development of such claims. The FDA approved the so-called qualified health claims for foods like nuts and olive oil for heart health, which is probably good advice, since healthy fats are not well understood by a generation who were told to avoid fats.

Qualified health claims set off a stream of comments from grocery associations, food police organizations, and food journalists (like I said, we love this stuff). To food manufacturers, the change in vernacular was a Pandora's box that would "provide food manufacturers with new incentives to develop and market new healthier-for-you products." For those who watch the grocery industry with a critical eye, the statement was an invitation backward to the days of the Tower of Babel, referring to the time before the NLEA, when unregulated health claims were rampant.

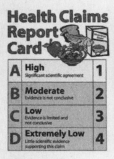
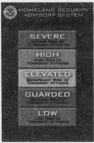

McClellan was quick to clarify that his statement was simply to introduce a new regulatory grading process that codes numerically and by color the level of scientific agreement for a qualified health claim. The coding looks a lot like John Ashcroft's Homeland Security terrorism codes. For instance, anything with a level A your mother would recommend. A purple-coded, level-B claim might be true, meaning there's a good chance you will get your money's worth. C is iffy. But be very wary of blue level D, the chances are extremely low the claim is substantiated, and the risk of wasting your money is high.

A consumer study released in October 2005 showed that even with this grading system, consumers perceived that B and C grades were more credible than level-A claims. The study suggested that shoppers are suspicious when they feel marketers are trying to influence them. Gee, really? It's not certain that this grading scheme will ever fly; Commissioner McClellan resigned before the system could be implemented, as did his successor, Commissioner Lester Crawford, two months after his Senate confirmation. In the summer of 2006, the idea reemerged. The FDA has not yet decided if qualified health claims will follow this report card format. Until then, the agency will review qualified health claims on a case-by-case basis.

The most recent qualified health claim petitions were for tomatoes and green tea, both for cancer claims. Tomatoes got a maybe and green tea was nixed. The approved language is so cautious that I'm not sure if expending the ink is worth the trouble or whether it's convincing enough to make me buy more tomatoes. You decide—here is the label:

> Very limited and preliminary scientific research suggests that eating one-half to one cup of tomatoes and/or tomato sauce a week may reduce the risk of prostate cancer. FDA concludes that there is little scientific evidence supporting this claim.

Processing the Meaning of Organic Processed Foods

While vast majorities were elated to see the final NOP released in October 2002, critics stewed. Voices of dissent were finally heard in a court case filed by Arthur Harvey, a Maine blueberry farmer and early opponent of the final rules. The suit cited that the NOP didn't comply with the original 1990 Organic Food Production Act (OFPA), the legislation the organic rules were founded on. The Harvey case summed up the displeasure of the organic purists over the fact that organically certified products could include synthetic ingredients (from a list of thirty-eight possibilities), as well as blanket approval for other non-organic ingredients. The NOP also gave some leeway when certain organic ingredients weren't available and allowed for nonorganic substitutions. In addition, food processing involves machinery and storage, which means even organic food processing relies on hundreds of substances (called noncontact food substances) to keep the equipment clean and the food safe. The Harvey court case argued that all of these practices exceeded the law's original intent.

Since the rules for organic certification were first approved, thousands of manufacturers have relied on these stipulations to increase the number of processed organic foods from a mere hundred to thousands. In time, the number of unapproved provisions increased, which maddened people like Harvey and fueled his desire to keep the case going long enough for a First Circuit Court judge in Boston to agree with his interpretation of the NOP laws.

At first glance, the case may not seem earth-shattering—but for the industry, it stopped them in their organic tracks. The decision could have forced farmers and manufacturers to throw out years of growing practices and product formulations and reinvent the organic wheel. The court ruling was nullified by quick action from the Organic Trade Association (OTA) with a rider attachment to an existing Agricultural Appropriations Bill—a move that was deemed by the Organic Consumers Association a "sneak attack" and a "dilution of the organic rules." In the manufacturers' opinion the OTA's lightning response simply kept things the way they had always been.

To understand the issues, let's look at organic certification rules. Organic products may be certified under three conditions—100% organic, organic, and made with organic ingredients. The Harvey court case threatened to downgrade at least 70% of the certified organic products to the lowest and least visible class. Here is what the rules allow for:

100% Organic: Must contain (excluding water and salt) only organically produced ingredients to carry the green and white symbol.
Organic: Must consist of at least 95% organically produced ingredients (excluding water and salt); the remaining 5% of the ingredients

can only come from a list of ingredients approved by an independent board.

Made with Organic Ingredients: Must contain at least 70% organic ingredients. Products in this category cannot use the organic symbol.

One provision from the Harvey case that held up was that manufacturers had to submit a list of all the nonorganic ingredients they relied on—if by January 2007 those ingredients were not on the national list, the product would no longer carry the organic symbol. There are still vocal organic food activists who say this isn't enough and that organic foods should be in the purest form possible.

FROZEN FOCACCIA AND SALAD DEBATE

Much of this debate harkens back to the days when few thought that a full spectrum of organic processed foods was even possible. Some believed that the modern methods of food manufacturing might lead to just another type of high-fat, low-quality, mediocre, commercial food production, rather than clean, unadulterated organic food—as nature intended.

Instead of rehashing boring court documents and arguments on each side of the organic fence, let's look at the issue of synthetics with this example. Say you invite your neighbor over for lunch. She lets herself in the back door with a plate of freshly baked organic chocolate-chip cookies (she's that kind of friend). Waiting at the table is a glass serving bowl (the one you borrowed from her) filled with layers of tender spring spinach and jumbo shrimp; a bottle of dressing sits alongside. As you flip the oven door shut with your foot and set a warm slab of onion and olive whole-wheat focaccia on the counter, she asks, "Is this all organic?"

Your neighbor knows your answer will be "yes." Are you telling the truth—an Abe Lincoln sort of honesty—or are you elaborating? The answer lies in whether you want to return to the days of healthy and chaste organic foods, which may be less than appetizing because they tend to spoil too quickly to make it to market, or you think the quality of organic foods in 2007 is a big improvement. Let's return to the menu to see what is at stake.

One of the fastest-growing organic food categories is bagged greens, such as lettuce and our lunch special, spinach. As you read in the produce chapter, food-borne bacteria—such as *E. coli*—thrive very agreeably on the tender leaves packed snugly inside the plastic bags. To retard the deadly microbes, the produce may be washed in a food-grade antibacterial solution or be exposed to carbon dioxide gas, which is why the bags often look like plastic blowfish. After packaging, the equipment is cleaned with approved disinfectants to prevent any trace microbes from multiplying into a lethal mass—there can be no detectable cleaning residues left on the machinery.

Perched atop the salad greens are U.S.-farmed organic jumbo shrimp. While shopping, you vaguely recalled reports about imported shrimp polluted with heavy metals and salmonella bacteria, as well as questions of whether there is such a thing as organic shrimp. Still, the organic brand seemed like the safest choice. (It's true that in April 2004 certification for organic shrimp was in jeopardy, but it was quickly restored by a temporary USDA ruling. Expect a final decision on the issue in the next few years.)

To dress the salad, you've chosen a favorite low-fat bottled dressing that contains the standard ingredients of oil, vinegar, flavorings, followed by xanthan gum and pectin to thicken and bind the liquids with the oil. Since lunch is with a close friend, you feel at ease and sop up the dressing with the whole-wheat focaccia. The texture is remarkably light—thanks to dough conditioners that give the whole grain the boost it needs to rise. To wash it all down, you have some grapefruit-flavored, Splenda-sweetened soda with your friend.

If one carefully examines the farming methods, the production practices, and the combination of ingredients in today's lunch and applies them to the Harvey court decision, the court ruling questioned the use of carbon dioxide to kill bacteria in the lettuce, disinfectants to clean machinery, and gums and emulsifiers to thicken the salad dressing. The other sector hardest hit by the proposed tighter restrictions would be frozen foods, especially frozen pizza and focaccia, because ascorbic acid (vitamin C) and calcium phosphates are used as dough conditioners and both are considered synthetic by organic standards. In addition, carbon dioxide is commonly used to reduce pest infestation in the grain silos that hold the wheat for the pizza and fo-caccia.

Technically, by organic standards, all of these ingredients and pro-cedures are considered synthetic, but don't let the word "synthetic" scare you. Among the synthetic ingredients approved by the NOSB, many are as familiar as baking soda in baked goods and iron in forti-fied cereals. There are another few hundred that are reserved for non-contact uses, to clean machinery and process food. There have been heated discussions as to whether to allow this list to include ingredi-ents like high-fructose corn syrup and alternative sweeteners in or-ganic foods. Even the mere suggestion has further fueled the opinion that organic foods should not include anything even remotely pro-cessed.

MILK AND COOKIE CRISIS

Back to lunch. Catching up on gossip, you dunk the chocolate-chip cookies in organic milk from a local dairy that recently converted to organic production, which brings up the last two issues: shortages of organic ingredients and feed standards for dairy herds. The cookies are sinfully thick with chocolate chips, although your neighbor has a secret—they came from a mix, made with organic whole-wheat and unbleached white flour (treated with CO_2), organic cane juice sugar (treated with lime), organic vanilla, baking soda, and baking powder (both technically synthetic ingredients)—see how pervasive this is?

If an organic ingredient is in short supply, such as the vanilla in the cookies, the manufacturer must prove to the organic certifier that it's not commercially available—a high price is not an excuse. For in-stance, organic vanilla supplies are often scarce due to damaging trop-ical storms, making this provision important. The court case could have severely limited which ingredients were open to the waiver.

The last issue remaining is organic milk. Perhaps you've noticed in your dairy case that organic milk supplies can't keep up with demand. Organic dairy farmers are pleading with other farmers to convert their herds to organic. It's a good problem to have. However, to hasten the transition from conventional to organic, a provision allowed cows to receive 20% nonorganic feed during the early phase of transition. In

April 2006, USDA regulators reviewed this practice and called for an end to it (see the dairy chapter).

Above all, the organic standards didn't come about in a vacuum. They were approved after more than a decade of collaboration among thousands of unlikely groups of people; many were business competitors and still more held very politically diverse opinions. That multiplicity is now emerging as clashes about semantics and lifestyle, precipitated by beliefs that foods produced by megacompanies like Pepsi and General Mills are not organic enough. Remember, the NOP provides *minimum* standards and anyone may exceed these rules and market products as such. However, there are safeguards and plenty of passionate people to protect against sneak attacks and reverse decisions that may indeed weaken the rules. Enjoy your organic lunch; the peace of mind is on me.

Labeling: More Is More, Less Is More

NUTRIENT CONTENT CLAIMS

These are recognizable by common words like "light," "free," and "enriched." These familiar words may have a slightly different meaning from what you hope; "free" isn't always completely free and "reduced" is only as good as the product's original formulation. It's not essential that you remember the exact meaning of each term, but be aware of the manner in which they are used.

FREE: Contains none or a negligible amount of the nutrient preceding the word "free." Sugar-free, for example, can contain less than 0.5g of sugar per serving (about .1 of a teaspoon). Saturated fat–free products may contain .5g or less of saturated fat and trans fats per serving and still carry the claim. If you consume a lot more than the suggested serving size, this food is no longer "free" of the given ingredient.

LOW: Products cannot contain more than a specific amount of the nutrient or ingredient in question, such as:
- Low sodium: no more than 140mg per serving size
- Very low sodium: no more than 35mg per serving size

- Low calorie: no more than forty calories per serving size
- Low fat: no more than 3g per serving size
- Low saturated fat: no more than 1g per serving size
- Low cholesterol: no more than 20mg per serving size.

Despite what you may have seen, there is no definition of low sugar or low carbohydrate. A definition is being worked out for the latter; until then, any low-carbohydrate claim can mean just about anything.

REDUCED OR LESS: Contains at least 25% less of a nutrient or calories than the regular product. If the referenced food is normally high in salt, sugar, or fat, particularly trans fats, the reduction may not be significant enough to be much healthier. The label must list the referenced food product, so compare the standard and the reduced values to make your judgment.

LIGHT (OR LITE): Has one-third fewer calories per serving than a comparable product, or 50% less fat or sodium per serving than a similar product. "Lite" can also mean the color or texture is lighter, such as "lite" olive oil or "light" brown sugar.

GOOD SOURCE: Provides between 10 and 19% of the DV of the nutrient being described.

HIGH, RICH IN, OR EXCELLENT SOURCE: Includes 20% or more of the DV for a nutrient.

MORE: Contains at least 10% more of the DV for a nutrient per serving than a comparison food.

LEAN: For meat, poultry, seafood, and game meats (fresh, frozen, or canned) that have less than 10g fat, less than 4g saturated fat, and less than 95mg cholesterol per standardized serving.

EXTRA LEAN: Meat, poultry, seafood, and game meats (fresh, frozen, or canned) that contain less than 5g fat, 2g saturated fat, and 95mg cholesterol per standardized serving.

HEALTHY: Meets the definition for low fat and saturated fat, contains no more than 60mg of cholesterol and 480mg of sodium per serving, and provides at least 10% of the DV for vitamin A, vitamin C, protein, calcium, iron, and fiber. This label is a good measure of a product that is low in fat and cholesterol but not sodium. If you must follow a low-sodium diet, the term "healthy" may fall short of your dietary constraints, since it allows for 480mg per serving and low-sodium foods cannot exceed 140mg per serving. This allowance was set to satisfy the needs of food manufacturers and meet the highest possible limits within the "healthy" range (see the sidebar on sodium at the end of the chapter).

AUTHORIZED HEALTH CLAIMS (FDA APPROVED, STRONG EVIDENCE)

Health claims for processed foods that need a nod from the FDA are those that connect food to a disease. Once marketers get ahold of health claims by adding vignettes and symbols (like cute little hearts), the claim might look different from the following FDA docket versions:

CALCIUM AND OSTEOPOROSIS: *"A diet adequate in calcium may help reduce the risk for osteoporosis, a degenerative bone disease."* Must contain 20% or more of the 200mg DV for calcium per serving and contain a form of calcium that is easily absorbed by the body.

FAT AND CANCER: *"A low-fat diet may help lower the risk for developing some types of cancer."* This only applies if the food is deemed low fat (no more than 3g per serving). However, for canned and frozen fish, poultry, and meat, the claim can be used as long as the food is extra-lean—5g of fat, less than 2g of saturated fat, and less than 95mg of cholesterol per serving.

SATURATED FAT, CHOLESTEROL, AND CORONARY HEART DISEASE: *"Diets low in saturated fat and cholesterol may lower blood cholesterol levels and reduce the risk for the development of CHD."* This claim has three criteria:
- Low saturated fat: 1g saturated fat or less per serving and 15% or less of calories from saturated fat. For a frozen or boxed meal, 1g saturated fat or lower and less than 10% of calories from saturated fat.
- Low cholesterol: 20mg cholesterol or less per serving; saturated fat content must be 2g or less in a serving.
- Low fat: less than 3g per serving.

FIBER-CONTAINING GRAIN PRODUCTS, FRUITS, AND VEGETABLES AND CANCER: *"Diets high in fiber and low in fat may reduce the risks for developing some types of cancer."* Contains the mentioned ingredients, is low fat (3g or less) and a good source of fiber, with no fortification (3–4g per serving).

FIBER-CONTAINING FRUITS, VEGETABLES, AND GRAINS AND CORONARY HEART DISEASE: *"Along with eating a diet low in fat, saturated fat, and cholesterol, fiber may help reduce blood cholesterol levels and the risk for developing heart disease."* Contains the mentioned ingredients and is low fat (3g or less), low in saturated fat (1g or less), and low in cholesterol (20g or less) and, without fortification, contains at least .6g soluble fiber per serving.

SODIUM AND HYPERTENSION: *"A low-sodium, low-salt diet may help to prevent the development of high blood pressure."* Product must have 140mg or less sodium per serving (see the sodium sidebar).

POTASSIUM AND HIGH BLOOD PRESSURE AND STROKE: *"Diets containing foods that are a good source of potassium and that are low in sodium may reduce the risk of high blood pressure and stroke."* Only for foods that are a good source of potassium (at least 350mg), low in total fat, saturated fat, and cholesterol, and low in sodium.

FRUITS AND VEGETABLES AND CANCER: *"Diets high in fruits and vegetables and low in fat may help reduce the risk for developing some types of cancer."* Fruits or vegetables low in fat (3g or less), with at least 500 IU vitamin A and 6mg vitamin C and 2.5g dietary fiber.

FOLATE OR FOLIC ACID AND NEURAL BIRTH DEFECTS: *"Healthful diets with adequate folate may reduce a woman's risk of having a child with neural tube defects."* Meets or exceeds 40mcg folic acid per serving. A serving cannot contain more than 100% of the DV for vitamins A or D because of potential risk to fetuses.

OMEGA-3 FATTY ACIDS: *"Supportive but not conclusive research shows that consumption of EPA and DHA omega-3 fatty acids may reduce the risk of coronary heart disease."* Foods must be low in cholesterol and low in saturated fat, which is why omega-3-enriched eggs may not carry this claim.

DIETARY SOLUBLE FIBER, FOUND IN WHOLE OATS AND PSYLLIUM SEED HUSK AND BARLEY (NEWEST ADDITION) AND HEART DISEASE: *"When* *included in a diet low in saturated fat and cholesterol, soluble fiber may lower blood cholesterol levels and lower the risk for heart disease."* The food must be low in fat (3g or less), saturated fat (1g or less), and cholesterol (20mg or less), and contain at least 0.75g of soluble fiber per serving. The fiber can come from whole oats, beta-glucan from oats, whole-grain barley, dry-milled barley ingredients, and psyllium seed husks (the same fibrous plant material used in products like Metamucil; however, it must be 1.7g of soluble fiber).

DIETARY SUGAR ALCOHOLS AND DENTAL CAVITIES: *"Frequent between-meal consumption of foods high in sugars and starches promotes tooth decay. The sugar alcohols in this food do not promote tooth decay"* or *"Does not promote tooth decay."* Meets the criteria for sugar-free (less than .5g per serving). The sugar alcohol can be xylitol, sorbitol, mannitol, maltitol, isomalt, lactitol, hydrogenated starch hydrolysates, hydrogenated glucose syrups, erythritol, or a combination of these.

SOY PROTEIN AND CORONARY HEART DISEASE: *"Diets low in saturated fat and cholesterol that include 25 grams of soy protein a day may reduce the risk of heart disease. One serving of [name of the food] provides _____ grams of soy protein."* Foods such as soy beverages, tofu, tempeh, soy-based meat alternatives, and baked goods must be low fat (3g or less), low saturated fat (1g or less), and low cholesterol (20mg or less). Whole soybeans, such as canned soybeans and soybean pods, called *edamame*, which are higher in fat, can carry the claim as long as no fat has been added.

PLANT STEROLS, STANOLS, AND CORONARY HEART DISEASE: *"Foods containing at least 0.65 grams per serving of plant sterol esters, eaten twice a day with meals for a daily total intake of at least 1.3 grams, as part of a diet low in saturated fat and cholesterol, may reduce the risk of heart disease. A serving of [name of the food] supplies _____ grams of plant sterol esters."* *"Diets low in saturated fat and cholesterol that include two servings of foods that provide a daily total of at least 3.4 grams of plant stanol esters in two meals may reduce the risk of heart disease. A serving of [name of the food] supplies _____ grams of plant stanol esters."* Studies show that 1.3g per day of plant sterol esters or 3.4g per day of plant stanol esters in the diet have a significant cholesterol-lowering effect. In order to qualify for this health claim, a food must contain at least 0.65g of plant sterol esters per serving or at least 1.7g of plant stanol esters per serving. The claim must specify that the daily dietary intake of plant sterol esters or plant stanol esters should be consumed in two servings eaten at different times of the day with other foods.

Remember the two-serving rule for this health claim. New foods are constantly being developed with plant sterol and stanols, but it may mean eating, for instance, plant-sterol margarine on your toast and a plant-sterol-enhanced granola bar for a snack.

QUALIFIED HEALTH CLAIMS (FDA APPROVED, LIMITED EVIDENCE)

These claims do not meet significant scientific agreement standards required by the FDA, but there is still limited evidence to support the statement. Expect to see more of these types of claims in the future. Both conventional foods and dietary supplements may display qualified health claims:

NUTS AND HEART DISEASE: *"Scientific evidence suggests but does not prove that eating 1.5 ounces per day of most nuts [such as name of specific nut] as part of a diet low in saturated fat and cholesterol may reduce the risk of heart disease."* The claim includes almonds, hazelnuts, peanuts, pecans, some pine nuts, pistachio nuts, and walnuts.

WALNUTS AND HEART DISEASE: *"Supportive but not conclusive research shows that eating 1.5 ounces per day of walnuts, as part of a low-saturated-fat and low-cholesterol diet, and not resulting in increased caloric intake, may reduce the risk of coronary heart disease."*

OMEGA-3 FATTY ACIDS AND CORONARY HEART DISEASE: *"Supportive but not conclusive research shows that consumption of EPA and DHA omega-3 fatty acids may reduce the risk of coronary heart disease."* Eligible foods are fresh, canned, and frozen fish and fish oil dietary supplements (the claim does not apply to flaxseed, because only limited amounts of its essential fatty acid, linolenic acid, are converted to EPA and DHA).

**MONOUNSATURATED FATTY ACIDS, OLIVE OIL, AND CORONARY HEART DIS-
EASE:** *"Limited and not conclusive scientific evidence suggests that
eating about 2 tablespoons of olive oil daily may reduce the risk of
coronary heart disease due to the monounsaturated fat in olive oil. To
achieve this possible benefit, olive oil is to replace a similar amount
of saturated fat and not increase the total number of calories you eat
in a day."*

DIETARY SUPPLEMENTS

- **Antioxidants and Cancer:** *"Some scientific evidence suggests
  that consumption of antioxidant vitamins may reduce the risk of
  certain forms of cancer. However, FDA has determined that this
  evidence is limited and not conclusive."*
- **Selenium and Cancer:** *"Selenium may reduce the risk of
  certain cancers. Some scientific evidence suggests that
  consumption of selenium may reduce the risk of certain forms of
  cancer. However, FDA has determined that this evidence is
  limited and not conclusive."*
- **B Vitamins and Vascular Disease:** *"As part of a well-
  balanced diet that is low in saturated fat and cholesterol, Folic
  Acid, Vitamin B_6, and Vitamin B_{12} may reduce the risk of
  vascular disease. FDA evaluated the above claim and found that,
  while it is known that diets low in saturated fat and cholesterol
  reduce the risk of heart disease and other vascular diseases, the
  evidence in support of the above claim is inconclusive."*
- **Phosphatidylserine and Cognitive Dysfunction and
  Dementia:** *"Consumption of phosphatidylserine* may reduce
  the risk of dementia in the elderly. Very limited and preliminary
  scientific research suggests that phosphatidylserine may reduce
  the risk of dementia in the elderly. FDA concludes that there is
  little scientific evidence supporting this claim."*
- **Folic Acid and Neural Tube Defects:** *"0.8mg folic acid in a
  dietary supplement is more effective in reducing the risk of
  neural tube defects than a lower amount in foods in common*

*Phosphatidylserine is sourced from soy.

form. FDA does not endorse this claim. Public health authorities recommend that women consume 0.4mg folic acid daily from fortified foods or dietary supplements or both to reduce the risk of neural tube defects."

CANNED AND FROZEN MISCELLANEOUS LABELS

Can Codes   Cans are stamped with a packing code for tracking during interstate commerce or rotating stock at the store and as an identifier for recalls. The letters and numbers refer to the date and time of manufacture and are not meant to be a use-by date.

If you do see a calendar date, it is a best-if-used-by date. High-acid canned foods such as tomatoes, grapefruit, and pineapple can be stored for twelve to eighteen months; low-acid canned foods such as meat, poultry, fish, and most vegetables will keep two to five years, as long as the can is in good condition.

Fresh(ly) Frozen   This is not a nutrient content claim, but it can be used for foods that are quickly frozen while still fresh. Canned foods have borrowed the term "freshly cut" to mean the same thing.

Flash Frozen   This quick freezing method takes place on fishing trawlers, allowing for seafood to be frozen within two hours of catch and in as little as three seconds. The seafood is packed and shipped frozen, held in subzero freezers, and never thawed.

Bottom Line

Within the inner aisles of the grocery store there is more clarity than in the days of Babel. The biggest drawback is that once you are faced with reading an actual food label, it's hard to tell whether a government agency approved or didn't approve the claim. Here is the general rule: Any statement that pairs a food with reducing the risk of a disease is a real, no-kidding health claim, such as sodium and hypertension or calcium and osteoporosis. *Unqualified claims,* categorized as A-level claims, aren't burdened with language that "qualifies" the level of scientific support.

A statement that measures the level of scientific support is a *qualified health claim*, such as "evidence suggests but does not prove" that nuts may reduce heart disease. You can always identify a qualified health claim by words such as "not conclusive," "limited," and "little scientific evidence."

There is one caveat to both unqualified and qualified health claims—none of these foods is a single magic bullet to better health. Perhaps the most widely promoted food with extraordinary health properties is soy. Health claims regarding soy, have been questioned lately, asking whether the bean is as magical as was once thought, because conflicting research is popping up questioning its role in preventing heart disease. Soy won't solve all your health problems; no food can justifiably make that claim. However, soy, as well as all the other foods that carry health claims, can be a part of a balanced, calorie-controlled, healthy diet—which collectively, in the long run, will reduce many common health problems. But none of them will overcome a poor diet and no exercise. Last, some of the foods with health claims are calorie dense, such as nuts, oils, and foods containing heart-healthy plant sterols, so don't overdo it.

Next in line are *nutrient content claims* like "no fat," "fortified," "reduced sugar," and "lite," which are used prolifically by 50% of food manufacturers. The most controversial are *structure/function* claims, which pit common sense against our hypochondriac inner souls by pairing claims with natural states of being—such as "may improve memory" or "maintaining healthy intestinal flora."

For decades the FDA was in a pressure cooker to approve the increasing number of health claims. The pro-labeling argument is that such terms point consumers in the right direction for better health, which can be true, but just as likely, the labels help sell more food. For me, if it's a healthy food already, the claim is a good reminder, such as the dietary guidance message for beans or fruits and vegetables. If a less-than-healthy food is simply enhanced, be careful. For instance, calcium-fortified frozen orange juice is a good choice—but calcium-fortified diet soda? Forget about it.

Last, while the green and white organic symbol may be under attack by individuals who prefer to live off the grid of conventional food manufacturing, it is more a lifestyle issue than one of food quality or safety. I remember the days when a moth might jump out of the bulk oat and flour bin at the health-food store. I also recall the frustration when I took the time to drive across town to the health-food store, past three conventional grocery stores, only to find what I wanted wasn't available. No thank you. I want to have my organic milk *and* cookies and eat them, too.

SALT WARNING

Canned and frozen vegetables don't get nearly the attention they deserve; they are a healthy and convenient option in our time-crunched lives. Canned and frozen vegetables and fruits are as nutritious as cooked fresh produce because they are processed soon after harvest. In some cases, they exceeded their raw counterparts for nutrients like lycopene and calcium in canned tomatoes.

The nutritional benefits and convenience trade-offs of canned and frozen can be undermined if the food contains too much salt, though. This applies not just for single foods like canned peas and corn but also for canned, frozen, and boxed meals.

Excessive sodium is one of the contributing factors for hypertension, a silent disease that affects as many as 65 million Americans. Research shows that it's not necessarily a heavy hand with the saltshaker that contributes to America's over consumption of salt—it's processed foods. The most sodium anyone should consume in one day is about 2,400mg, or no more than a teaspoon. Americans over fifty should consume about 1,500mg because of increased risk of hypertension, stroke, and osteoporosis, since sodium leaches calcium from the bones.

In June 2006, the American Medical Association (AMA) called for Americans to break free of our love affair with salt. To remind us of our unhealthy relationship, the AMA is suggesting that foods with high sodium levels be labeled as such with a saltshaker bearing the word

(continued)

"high" and red exclamation points to get our attention. Foods with more than 480mg sodium per serving would be considered high salt.

Small amounts of sodium can add up quickly when you are eating processed foods, even if you try to eat healthy. Here is how salt shakes out in this example of a relatively healthy daily menu. Breakfast: instant oatmeal with brown sugar cinnamon (325mg), ½ cup juice-packed canned peaches (5mg); lunch: turkey sandwich on whole-wheat bread (1,800mg), ½ cup tomato soup (713mg); dinner: green salad with fat-free bottled Italian salad dressing (280mg), broiled chicken breast with a pinch of salt (150mg), ½ cup canned corn with ½ tsp. butter (220mg); dessert: mint chip no-sugar, light ice cream (50mg). Are you ready? The grand total is 3,543mg of sodium; that's without any snacks.

Now keep the basic menu the same with some small changes, such as: regular oatmeal (2mg), lower-sodium roast turkey (430mg), low-salt tomato soup (90mg), and a green salad with homemade vinegar EVOO dressing (0mg). The sodium level measures out at 947mg, or less than half a teaspoon, which leaves room for a pinch here and there to season your food.

Even if you shake a few grains on your food, the added salt won't come close to what is hidden in processed foods. Manly-men frozen dinners are big culprits, with as much as an entire day's sodium intake in one meal. Or for petite appetites, one small meal from a healthy-sounding brand might be considered two portions by the manufacturer—the whole meal could easily meet half your day's sodium allotment.

It's hard to deny that salt makes food taste better—it brightens flavors like no other spice in the kitchen. With increasing reliance on restaurants and processed foods in our diets, we have unknowingly steadily raised American salt intake to unhealthy levels. Our foods have gotten so salty without our realizing it that the Center for Science in the Public Interest and the AMA want sodium to be considered an additive, which would have tighter controls than it does in its current status as an ingredient "generally recognized as safe." The center's stance is so ardent, the consumer watchdog group is suing the FDA to push the agency toward some sort of salt regulation.

For now, pay close attention to salt levels in processed foods. Don't rely on the front of the box, bottle, or can for a hint. Even the word "healthy" can lead you astray, because it allows for as much as 480mg of sodium per serving—a low-sodium label is a better measure (140mg). Also, be aware of foods that don't necessarily have a salty reputation, like canned crushed tomatoes. This kitchen staple can vary among brands by a few hundred milligrams—Hunt's 350mg, Contadina 150mg, and Muir Glen 100mg.

The Canned Food Alliance recommends rinsing canned vegetables before cooking to reduce the sodium levels by as much as 40%. The last word on salt is to remember that sodium isn't always labeled in easily recognizable words, so look for monosodium glutamate, sodium citrate, sodium nitrate, sodium phosphate, sodium saccharin, and even baking soda and baking powder in baked goods.

CHAPTER 11

Social Unrest:
A Wake-Up Call for the Coffee and Tea Industry

Illegal Immigration: The Coffee Industry's Pawns

Each spring break my teenage son packs up for a trip. It's not what you think; instead of a beach resort with drinking and wild women, he goes to some of the most underserved areas of this country, the inner city of Los Angeles or poor communities along the Mississippi River, to work in shelters and poverty-stricken communities. In the spring of 2005, he went to the U.S.-Mexican border with his church.

One of their projects was to walk the border in Mexico and clean up trash and place water along this highway of humanity for illegal crossings. Amid the tuna cans and water and beer bottles, they came upon a few dozen people sitting less than ten feet from the mangled barbed-wire fence that marks the line in the sand between Mexico and the United States. Pastor Glenn Perica described the scene as an "odd game of chess." From his vantage point, at six feet, eight inches tall, he could see the red flags marking water stations set up by humanitarian aid groups to the south; toward the north the U.S. horizon was dotted with border patrol towers and vehicles.

The Mexicans sat like pawns in the brittle, sunburned desert while kings and knights waited for their next move on the opposing side of the game board. The two groups approached each other with trepidation. This was the same week the Minutemen Militia began their quest to prevent the nightly influx of illegal immigrants—tension was high. As the church group's guide explained to the Mexicans that their chances of crossing undetected were slim, a blast of air from a border patrol helicopter tumbled down on the crowd, spraying sand in all directions.

Perica and my teenage son lay prostrate in the Sonoran Desert while the immigrants hid their faces from cameras in the aircraft overhead. As the helicopter veered away, a handful of reporters and documentary filmmakers, with more cameras rolling, entered the scene from nowhere, recording a capsule of time that spoke volumes about the complexity of the crisis.

That night, my son's youth group prayed, talked, and prayed again. Their hearts were broken, their minds numb, from the grief and destitution around them. They also knew that back home some would interpret their chance meeting with the Mexicans as offering assistance. The problems and the solutions were too enormous for them to grasp.

A day later, they found hope in a tiny two-room coffee cooperative called Just Coffee, tucked away on a dirt road in Agua Prieta, the Mexican sister city to Douglas, Arizona. One pound of coffee at a time, the company seeks to mend years of economic damage by paying co-op coffee farmers in Salvador Urbina, Chiapas, a fair price and handing out free business advice on how to compete in an unforgiving coffee marketplace.

Just Coffee's success is largely due to a higher power, since the company's business mentors and clients are from American churches. The company estimates that if they sold coffee on the world market the thirty-five coffee-farming families would collect about $31,000, but as a free market co-op they recorded about $350,000 of sales in 2004. For me, it hits home when I see the name of the Chiapas farmer on my bag of coffee; this month it's Elifa Cifuentes L.

Are There Clouds in Your Coffee?

The predicament of illegal immigration has expanded beyond the headlines, hospitals, and schools in Southwestern and Western communities. It's now a hot button for the presidential election and a tense topic for watercooler discussions; even the high school in my town was featured in major news outlets when the principal banned flags because of student-led immigration protests. Many who lament over the problem fail to see that one of the many initial causes is as close and as dear as their morning cup of coffee.

As recently as a decade ago, Mexican coffee farmers made an adequate living in the highlands of Southern Mexico, until global coffee prices plunged to a hundred-year low. The steep drop came in 1989, after U.S. and Mexican governments decided to forgo a long-standing agreement, the International Coffee Agreement, which maintained stable prices at about $1.20 to $1.40 per pound. Decision makers knew that for too long the coffee marketplace hung by the bootstraps of a convoluted, government-controlled quota system that needed changing.

Unfortunately for the poorest of the lot—the farmer—the policy change was abrupt. Economic forecasters could have written the script blindfolded; prices fell steeply below production costs, and stored coffee flooded the surplus market. On the heels of deregulation, the World Bank helped Vietnam enter the already-glutted coffee market, further undercutting prices down the nibs. To add injury, Brazil, the largest coffee-growing country, replaced ice-damaged coffee trees with higher-yield varieties, further inundating the glutted supplies.

Few people from the coffee-growing regions thought about leaving their hometowns prior to the coffee crisis. Given the choice of starve or move, thousands of desperate growers gave up their land and headed north. Some sought work in large Mexican cities; others risked crossing the border. Coffee was Mexico's second largest commodity behind oil, ranking Mexico as the fourth-largest coffee producer on the planet. Now, as you well know, the imported American dollar is Mexico's second-largest commodity.

Since the late 1990s, migration rates from coffee-growing regions such as Chiapas and Veracruz jumped from last on the list of thirty-one Mexican states to near the top. The ripple sent rings of poverty southward, forcing as many as 600,000 coffee bean pickers from neighboring Central America to follow close behind. Now Mexico has its own immigration problem on its southern border. Coffee grows only in regions between the Tropics of Cancer and Capricorn in Africa, India, South and Central America, and the Caribbean, historically poor regions that tip easily with deep cuts in income and employment.

If Immigration Is the Question,
Is Fair Trade the Answer?

If the border situation can be compared to a high-powered game of chess, the coffee industry is easily an unfair game of Monopoly. While American coffee wholesalers maneuver profitably around the jagged ups and downs in the market, coffee farmers are handed weighted dice that repeatedly force them back to Go without collecting $200. For many years, the only hope was to draw a card from the Community Chest called fair trade.

What few realize is that for four dollars a day—the cost of a pound of canned coffee—a small coffee farmer will have worked an entire day to pick 200 pounds of coffee cherries, or about fifty pounds of finished beans. He will reap only $.10 to $.30 per pound of the retail price, even though it costs as much as $.60 per pound to cover production costs. The remaining money is paid out to the mills, shippers, exporters and importers, roasters, wholesalers, marketers, and retailers.

The next time you hear media reports about how Sara Lee, Procter & Gamble, Nestlé, and Kraft, which buy more than 60% of this country's coffee, are being forced to raise coffee retail prices, don't feel sorry for them. First, they paid for the coffee long before any unexpected price hikes, and second, profits among U.S. coffee wholesalers and packagers are more than adequate. Ten years ago, U.S. coffee retail sales topped $30 billion, with farmers receiving $10 billion. Today retail sales are more than double at $70 billion, but farmers see less than $8 billion, so profits are far from dismal on this Park Place side of the game board.

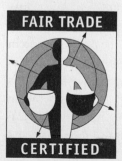

Fair trade seeks to overcome some of these inequities by guaranteeing a set price to member co-ops of $1.26 per pound ($1.41 for organic). On the few occasions when the market price exceeds that of fair trade, farmers receive the world market price and a $.05 premium.

The internationally used Fair Trade Certified label guarantees that prices, working conditions, and wages meet the standards set by the Fairtrade

Labelling Organization (FLO) in Bonn, Germany. TransFair USA certifies fair trade coffee imports into this country.

The first U.S. fair trade coffee seller was Equal Exchange, founded in 1986. The company sells to grocers and directly to consumers, including as many as 3,400 churches through its faith-based programs. Since its inception, more than twenty other American companies have taken up the cause, such as Global Exchange, Café Campesino, Dean's Beans, and Green Mountain. There are currently 221 Fair Trade Certified co-ops, representing more than 800,000 farmers and their families worldwide.

Is Fair Trade Fair?

Staunch supporters of open markets have described fair trade as an expensive and inefficient charity organization, citing that the market will right itself when supplies match demand. To do so, farmers must diversify to keep supplies down.

In a well-connected, well-orchestrated, modernized industry, this might be possible. However, the coffee industry is a hodgepodge of more than 25 million workers, living in the poorest regions of the world, often on isolated plots of land of no more than five to ten acres. Fair trade doesn't solicit farms into forming co-ops, like an organized union would; instead it offers services to farms that have already formed a co-op or wish to consolidate into a collective business.

The pessimistic argument against fair trade misses the mark—why should today's coffee farmers accept prices that importers paid during our great-grandparents' era? "The coffee market doesn't mandate fair wages," says Rodney North, spokesperson for Equal Exchange. "For instance, we have to pay our own coffee warehouse workers in the U.S. an acceptable wage, but for some reason the coffee industry draws a line at the border," he says. "Fair trade creates a system that is better connected and offers a sufficient wage appropriate for today's retail coffee prices."

There is no free ride in fair trade. Farmers who agree to fair trade have to meet their share of the bargain. "Joining a co-op takes work and effort, such as self-governance, good business practices, environmental and quality control measures," North says. There are coffee farmers who prefer not to deal with the extra work in exchange for a higher price, but they benefit vicariously, since the premiums reach well beyond the borders of the farm. "For instance, if the co-op decides to use fair trade premiums to pave a road into town or build a health clinic, everyone in the village uses the road or the clinic, not just the fair trade farmers," says Haven Bourque, spokesperson for TransFair USA.

The system doesn't just pay more for coffee, it assists with prefinancing, debt assistance, organic farming training, and marketing education to comprehend the North American and E.U. marketplace, North says. Fair trade coffee farmers also say that family life is stable and they feel a renewed pride in coffee farming—traits they lost during the coffee crisis. This hardly sounds like an international freebie welfare scheme.

There are signs that conventional supermarket coffee suppliers are making small concessions to fair trade. At the request of its shareholders, Procter & Gamble launched a fair trade Millstone brand, called Mountain Moonlight. Sara Lee brands Chock full o'Nuts and Chase & Sanborn sell fair trade coffee to hospitals and colleges, not grocery stores at this time. Kraft and Nestlé haven't yet budged on the issue (Nestlé introduced a fair trade brand in the E.U.). "The challenge is getting into the mainstream marketplace," says Bourque. "If soccer moms living in the furthest reaches of Iowa are willing to pay for fair trade coffee at the grocery store," she says, "then consumer empowerment alone will increase sales dramatically." That day may be closing in. As of this writing, Wal-Mart is exploring suppliers of Fair Trade coffee for its grocery stores.

Fair Trade, No Longer the Only White Horse in Town

The "feel good" story of fair trade has some limitations. Co-ops, like Just Coffee, survive very well outside the fair trade market. Their success has to do with similar governing principles to fair trade, such as democratic decision making, sound marketing plans, and control over distribution. Although coffee drinkers with a conscience upped sales of fair trade coffee in 2003 by 91% to 18.7 million pounds, on average, most Fair Trade Certified growers are lucky to sell 20 to 30% of their coffee as fair trade. The remaining coffee is sold to importers in the shaky commodities market and specialty coffee market, if the quality meets the mark. The Just Coffee co-op is able to sell *all* their coffee for a fair price.

On the one hand, in the early years of fair trade many specialty coffee buyers felt like the program was a type of socially conscious extortion. The quality wasn't on par with what many specialty coffee companies were seeking. The complaint was that fair trade pressured them to buy poor-quality coffee at a higher price.

On the other hand, fair trade supporters have accused specialty coffee companies, such as Starbucks, that sell some but not all fair trade coffee, of profiting by clinging to the coattails of fair trade without being brave enough to wear the uniform. In their defense, Starbucks is the biggest single U.S. buyer of fair trade coffee, exceeding more than 11.5 million pounds in 2005.

For Starbucks and other specialty coffee retailers it's a matter of quality coupled with volume. "From the Starbucks perspective, we are known for customer experience and a huge part of that is quality," says Diana Reid, Starbucks public affairs manager. Even fair trade experts admit that early on quality was a problem. Now, however, the world's leading tasting experts often unknowingly select fair trade coffee in cupping competitions over non–fair trade brands.

Volume and control over the cumbersome supply chain are the biggest obstacles to companies like Starbucks. Reining in the millions of remote coffee farmers to meet a large company's brand image of consistent taste and quality is like herding butterflies from five continents with one net. This is one reason that Starbucks relies on a blend of farms, small and large, including some that may not meet fair trade parameters. Coffee farms that hire labor, even one employee, don't qualify for fair trade, some farms are just too large, and still others are run by tribal governance, as in Africa, rather than Western-style democratic cooperatives. Few and far between are the coffee farmers who have the knowledge of how to market and negotiate with the specialty coffee brokers for themselves. "Fair trade is a good thing, but we don't want to discriminate against larger coffee farmers or farms that don't qualify for fair trade," says Reid. "In the broader scope, we are concerned about the entire coffee chain."

The philanthropic deeds of such conspicuous corporations aren't exactly equal to those of Robin Hood legends, but do they and other specialty coffee wholesalers deserve the bruises? Starbucks is known for paying coffee farmers well, as is the specialty coffee industry as a whole ($1.20 or more per pound, which is sometimes triple the price on the New York Coffee Exchange).

Perhaps these companies' only true fault is bad timing. In the early years, when Starbucks' brand awareness grew and profits mounted, the coffee industry was crumbling into a fine powder. It wasn't until consumer awareness about fair trade gained momentum and customers realized that their daily double vanilla latte contributed significantly to specialty coffee houses' profit margins to the detriment of farmers, that companies like Starbucks began to seriously look inward.

The rub is, as North says, "there are at least 54 different ways to get coffee to market." When any non–fair trade coffee seller advertises the price they pay for coffee, the underlying question is: Where is that money going—to an importer, a broker, or directly to the farmer? North asks. There is no one answer, since coffee buyers rely on all of these players to buy coffee, unlike in fair trade, which leaves out the middlemen.

Even this is changing—the Starbucks way. Starbucks is about consistency of image, brand, products, and customer service. The company is so good at branding they even have us speaking a new language—"tall, skinny, no whip, caramel *macchiato*, please." Which is why it's not surprising that they have their own farmer support program—one they control from bean to cup. Starbucks buys almost 25% of its coffee through a preferred supplier program called Coffee and Farmer Equity (CAFE). The CAFE program pays a fair price and assists with finances and community outreach programs, provided the growers meet Starbucks' quality and taste standards. By 2007, the company plans to purchase all of its coffee from CAFE and fair trade suppliers (the actual numbers were not available at press time).

Time will tell whether the scope and scale of Starbucks' CAFE program match or exceed those of fair trade. Bourque and North agree that fair trade practices have jump-started the overall coffee market by leveraging higher prices and challenging specialty coffee companies to promote positive change. If nothing else, the success of the fair trade coffee movement has prompted other nonprofits to promote their own various causes within the coffee industry, such as Coffee Corps, which teaches Rwandan coffee growers how to improve the quality of their crop and negotiate for higher prices. Coffee Kids funds education and health care, as well as provides training for jobs outside the coffee industry.

The true test is the commercial coffee market. For all the slingshots aimed across the coffee bar at Starbucks, the commercial canned coffee industry needs to be held more accountable. The biggest changes will come about only if we, the consumers, chink away bean by bean at their profits by purchasing coffee from suppliers who place the interests of the farmers prominently.

Now that activist groups have raised awareness about the issue, the collective dollar will be more powerful than boycotts and protests to promote change. "It's important that fair trade coffee promoters not come across as a bunch of crazy hippies," says Bourque. "We aren't going to break the windows at Starbucks and make progress," she says.

Coffee Labels

The coffee industry is void of any regulated terms, except the word "coffee." Manufacturers aren't required to tell you the type of bean or where it comes from. With the exception of Fair Trade, organic, and a few environmental labels, this industry is marked by illustrative and exotic descriptions that sound like an Ernest Hemingway novel— "leathery tobacco with undercurrents of tart, refreshing pie cherries." Bowing to competition from the specialty market, the commercial canned coffee sector has also opened up their thesaurus for descriptive terms. But be aware that there are no hard and fast rules for the labels and marketing vernacular.

COFFEE GRADE AND ROAST LABELING

Arabica and Robusta   There are more than two dozen species of coffee trees, a relative of the gardenia, but all you need to remember is Arabica and Robusta. The best quality Arabica beans are grown in mountain elevations on shaded, terraced hillsides and handpicked by nimble-footed workers. Lower-elevation Arabica is next in line, followed by Robusta beans, which are machine harvested and taste bitter, and therefore cannot be consumed alone. They account for about 30% of the world market and are used in instant coffee and in blends for canned coffee brands and espresso blends.

Most of the Robusta beans are grown in Asia and Brazil and fetch a dismal price, half that of Arabica beans. If a coffee ingredient label says 100% pure coffee, with no delineation between Arabica and Robusta, expect that at least 30% of the grounds to be Robusta.

Specialty Grade Coffee   Coffee-tasting experts, called cuppers, use their sensitive taste buds to identify coffee's unique qualities of fragrance (the smell of beans after grinding), aroma (the smell of ground beans after steeping in water), taste, nose (the vapors released by the coffee in the mouth), and body (the feel of the coffee on the tongue). For the educated taster, the distinctions stand out like the difference between water and wine; for the rest of us, it's a bit trickier.

Generally grocery department managers divide the coffee aisle into two distinct departments, commercial canned brands and specialty. Specialty beans are sold in bags or in bulk. The beans are larger than lower grades and have the fewest defects (broken beans, insect damage, and debris) and are void of quakers, which are notoriously stubborn beans that refuse to roast into a dark color. Canned coffee has more defects, which is why it is preground.

French, Italian, Viennese, American   Despite their names, these terms refer to the intensity of the roast, not the country of origin. Coffee beans are roasted at between 375 and 425 degrees Fahrenheit for ninety seconds to fifteen minutes. As the beans roast, the acidity declines, but bitterness increases. Talented roasters know the precise moment when the bean will exude a full-bodied flavor. If high-quality coffee beans are roasted beyond their limits, the aromas and flavor components will break down, though the overroasting can also remove flaws in poorer-quality beans.

Roasting verbiage varies from supplier—in order of lightest to darkest roasts look for American, Viennese, Italian, and French or light brown, medium brown, and dark brown. Medium roast coffees have the fullest flavor.

Sumatran, Kenyan, Mexican, Columbian, and So On In general, if you see country names outside Europe, located near the equator, this is a good indicator of where the beans were grown, such as India, Ethiopia, Jamaica, or Guatemala. Some barristers—the owners/servers at your favorite specialty coffee shop—will also add a city, landmark, region, estate, or cooperative name to further pinpoint the coffee's home turf.

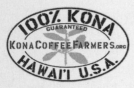

Kona Coffee This Hawaiian-grown coffee is protected by an active nonprofit association of coffee growers, called the Kona Coffee Farmers Association. Kona coffees are graded from highest to lowest coffee as extra fancy, fancy, No. 1, and prime, respectively. Kona coffee farmers and processors won a million-dollar lawsuit against the coffee company Kona Kai, which was indicted for relabeling bags of Latin American coffee as Kona. Authentic Kona coffee is grown only in the Kona region on the island of Hawaii. After roasting, the average retail price for 100% Kona coffee is forty-six to fifty-two dollars per pound, so don't be misled by blends that use only 10% Kona coffee.

Blended Coffee Commercial coffee roasters rely on blending a variety of beans to control cost and taste from batch to batch. Since coffee prices are extremely volatile and supplies are unwieldy, blenders deal with an array of beans from different regions with one goal in mind—consistent taste. For instance, a breakfast blend isn't made from any one type of bean, from any single region; it usually denotes a medium roast with a smooth taste.

Some coffee blends mix a rarer specialty coffee with a lower grade and name the coffee based on the higher-quality coffee. For instance, a Jamaican blend will contain some coffee from the island, considered one of the world's best, though the rest is a blend of beans from other regions of the world.

Espresso   If "What is espresso?" were a multiple-choice question, the answer would be "all of the above." The term "espresso" refers to (1) the way the coffee is ground, (2) a brewing method, and (3) the blend of beans. In Italian *espresso* means "fast," and everything about espresso is fast: Water is forced through the finely ground beans in about fifteen seconds, creating a thick, velvety cup that is meant to be consumed with gusto, rather than sipped like a frothy, milky cappuccino.

Espresso aficionados ponder the perfect *crema*, the froth on the top of the espresso. It's a tricky combination of the right Arabica and Robusta bean blend, extraction time, and water temperature—ask your favorite barrister for the instructions.

Flavored Coffee   "You can get every other flavor except coffee-flavored coffee! They got mochaccino; they got chocaccino, frappaccino, rappaccino, Al Pacino, what the f***." Denis Leary's famous quip about coffee says it all. Somewhere in the past decade Americans lost interest in coffee-flavored coffee and took a liking to ice-cream parlor tastes like chocolate, vanilla, and hazelnut. Flavored coffees are made by adding liquid flavoring to medium or dark roast coffee; unfortunately, there aren't any chocaccino or Al Pacino coffee trees.

Decaffeinated Coffee   Described by the caffeine dependent as the perfect cup of "Why Bother," decaf coffee is a growing trend, especially as the boomer generation ages and is beleaguered by sleep problems, heart palpitations, and caffeine jitters. As much as 20% of American coffee drinkers resort to decaf at one time or another.

Decaffeination removes 97% of the caffeine from green coffee beans in four ways: with the chemical solvent methylene chloride, with the naturally occurring solvent ethyl acetate (found in apples, peaches, and pears), with water and charcoal filters (Swiss water method), or with carbon dioxide. Methylene chloride is the same chemical banned from hairsprays because of ozone pollution. It's still FDA approved for coffee, though, because methylene chloride burns away at temperatures of only 104 degrees Fahrenheit—coffee roasting exceeds this by at least 300 degrees.

In 2003, researchers in Brazil used natural plant-breeding techniques to grow decaffeinated Arabica coffee beans. In addition, researchers in Japan have developed a GM coffee bean with 70% less caffeine. The Japanese-bred GM bean may beat the Brazilian non-GM bean to the market by a few years; there is no word on whether the FDA will allow GM labeling.

Decaf beans are weaker than fully leaded beans because the soaking and steaming they are put through make the beans difficult to roast. To compensate, ask your favorite coffee shop which varieties have less caffeine, such as African and Guatemalan beans, and blend them in a one-to-two ratio with a good-quality decaffeinated bean. Arabica beans contain about 1.5% caffeine, Robusta 2.5%, so switching to Arabica beans can reduce your caffeine consumption.

ECO-FRIENDLY, SOCIALLY CONSCIOUS LABELS

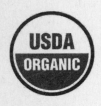

USDA Organic Certified   For many small coffee farmers pesticide use is not even on their radar screen, not because they are any less concerned about conservation than other farmers—they simply can't afford to buy the chemicals. This means that much of the small-estate coffee industry is pesticide free by default. Fair trade certifiers and specialty coffee field advisers use this advantage to help small farmers get organically certified or at least dissuade them from bending to pressure from chemical companies to use the deadliest of chemicals, known as the dirty dozen. Eighty-five percent of fair trade coffee is organic.

Should you worry about pesticides in coffee? Not as much for yourself as the farmer. Here's why: Two coffee beans hide deep within the pulp and skin of a coffee cherry, which is dried or soaked to remove the outer coatings. Then the green beans are fermented or soaked, dried, and roasted at temperatures exceeding 400 degrees Fahrenheit. Studies show that this brutal process reduces any pesticide residue to insignificant amounts.

Even though the beans may be free of pesticide residues, there is an altruistic reason to buy organic coffee—it improves the lives of coffee growers, their families, and the surrounding community by reducing groundwater contamination and pesticide exposure, especially for vulnerable children and workers who lack the literacy skills to read the directions properly and understand the dangers.

   Shade-Grown, Rainforest, and Bird Friendly Agriculture, the art and science of cultivating the land, has a bad habit of manipulating Mother Nature to suit the needs of man, rather than vice versa. For coffee harvesting, this meant increasing production by ripping out acres and acres of shade trees that naturally grew alongside coffee trees.

Farmers converted shade-loving coffee plants to sun worshipers in hopes that sun-grown coffee could pull them out of their financial woes. International development programs dumped more than $80 million in a twenty-year period to help growers learn more about the high-tech advances of sun-grown coffee. By the early 1990s, nearly 40% of previously shade-grown coffee was converted to sun coffee varieties.

It's never a good idea to fool Mother Nature, and coffee is no exception. In time agriculturists learned that sun-grown coffee didn't meet their expectations. The fields required costly fertilizer to make up for the missing nutrients in rich forest beds; sun coffee trees had shorter life spans than shade species by as much as seventy-five years, and with no trees there were no birds. Worse yet, sun-grown coffee commanded weaker global prices and the trees that used to provide alternative crops for income, such as tropical fruits and wood for fuel, were gone.

Various conservation groups took notice and began to promote shade-grown and conservation-friendly certified coffee. Rainforest

Alliance, Bird Friendly Coffee, and the National Wildlife Federation each play a role in this arena. The Rainforest Alliance certifies more than 50,000 farms for conservation growing methods. A recent certification is Juan Valdez–branded coffee. Products that bear the symbol are guaranteed to be beneficial to wildlife, farmers, and local communities. The seal is on coffee, bananas, paper, and even guitars.

The Smithsonian Migratory Bird Center certifies Bird Friendly Coffee on eleven farms in Colombia, Guatemala, Mexico, and Peru. The coffee must be grown under either rustic shade trees (naturally occurring) or planted shade trees. The National Wildlife Federation promotes a similar agenda as other bird-friendly certifiers. They are partnering with the Green Mountain coffee wholesaler to brand coffee that is fair trade, shade grown, and organic.

By the very character of their mission there is some overlap between these groups. For instance, all have an expectation of a shade-grown environment, making them all bird friendly. However, the Rainforest Alliance certification is larger in scope and breadth, and the group's main focus is to educate farmers about alternatives to destructive farming methods that lead to erosion and polluted water runoff.

The caveat is that not all coffee-growing regions need additional shade from trees. For example, in Costa Rica cloud cover offers more than adequate shade and additional trees would put the crops at risk for disease. So while it's rare to find shade-grown Costa Rican coffee, that's not an indicator of poor conservation practices.

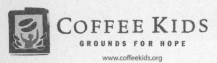

Coffee Kids Coffee Kids is a nonprofit organization that partners with nongovernmental community organizations in Latin America to create education, health-care, training, and microenterprise programs for coffee farmers and their families. The aim is to assist in the development of alternative income sources so adult family members can make money outside the volatile coffee industry, thus providing a stable home environment for families, free from the demands and disruption of migration. Although the organization admits they cannot entirely stop coffee workers from migrating during the harvesting season, Coffee Kids seeks to provide alternatives so children can stay in school and families have a year-round supplemental income to coffee harvesting.

Fairly Traded   When fair trade coffee activists garnered the attention of the media, some in the specialty coffee industry were put off by the negative attention, especially since much of the exploitation came as a result of inexpensive commercial coffee sales, not the sales of high-quality beans. To counter the attacks, words like "fairly traded coffee" were added to package descriptions.

The specialty coffee industry generally pays equal or above fair trade prices, if the quality warrants it. The big difference is that unless the wholesaler buys directly from the farmer, which is difficult, some of the money may go to the importer and a dozen other middlemen, peeling away pennies of profit from the farmer. If you care about this issue, make certain that the farmer is paid directly.

Descriptions on the package may also say the company offers economic incentives for better standards of living. It's hard to measure the scope of these programs from a label. The company may well have a comprehensive program that pays the farmer more money, assists with low-cost loans, and partners with social program agencies—or it may be limited in scope. If such efforts are important to you, take the time to learn more about the program.

One last warning: Fair trade coffee shouldn't cost much more than a standard house brand of specialty coffee. I took a survey of coffee shops and grocers in my area and found one specialty retailer and a grocery store selling fair trade at three dollars more per pound than other retailers. A letter is on the way reminding them that unless the farmers are getting that extra few dollars (which they aren't), exploitation doesn't make for good business practices.

Sustainable   This is perhaps the most widely abused term in the coffee business. The definition depends on what area of the industry you most sympathize with —birds, the environment, fair wages, community stability—or the coffee industry as a whole. While each niche is a noble cause, the International Coffee Organization (ICO) is undertaking the task of developing a wide-reaching definition of sustainability.

Minds met, committees were formed, and reports were generated by the ICO in 2004 to begin working toward a sustainable coffee industry. The two basic objectives, the report said, are "harmony between man and nature, implying respect for the planet's ecological limits; and harmony among human beings or, in other words, a measure of social cohesion." We can only hope the ICO will borrow the best features from successful examples within fair trade, specialty coffee, organic, shade-grown, and kid-friendly programs.

My Cup of Tea

Cowboy coffee, made from soaking grounds in boiled water, has been a rich staple of cowboy lore, especially in my adopted home state of Colorado. I believed every word of it until a friend and expert in Western food history, Holly Arnold Kinney (owner of The Fort restaurant, Morrison, Colorado), enlightened me. Cowboys almost certainly drank more tea than coffee, she said. Coffee was hard to come by, but tea was easily available from Asians working on the railroads. Compressed tea cakes, as hard as bricks, weighed little and stored easily in battered leather saddlebags (tea cakes are still available in specialty tea stores). The image sticks in my mind whenever I sip tea on my porch with an eye toward the Rocky Mountains to the west.

Until the late 1800s American ranch hands and city folk alike drank strong black Chinese tea. When the Chinese rebuked the British tea traders' practice of paying for tea with opium, the English looked to colonial India, which is now the world's largest tea-producing country. Eastern Africa also grows a good supply of high- and moderate-quality teas.

All tea comes from the *Camellia sinensis* plant, related to the camellia. The best teas are made from the uppermost bud and the two youngest leaves, which are harvested during the flushing, or sprouting, season. After harvest, the leaves are dried and fermented, a process in which enzymes lurking within tea leaves work their magic to transform the bitter plant into an astringent leaf perfect for a brisk cold drink or hot cup of tea. The dry leaves are sorted into grades such as whole leaf, broken leaf, cut, fannings, and dust. The latter three are used in tea bags.

Tea is known worldwide for its flavor and health properties, which come from essential oils and polyphenols within the leaves. The caffeine in tea is twice that of coffee, but since we use much less tea per cup than coffee the jitters are less noticeable. Tea also has a countering calming component, an amino acid called L-theanine, which is particularly notable in green tea.

Tea packaging is considered the fashion plate of the food world. In fact, cosmetic packaging experts move easily into the tea industry, since the customers are from the same pool of women. "It's all about packaging," says Maria Uspenski, proprietor of the Tea Spot teahouse and retail tea line in Boulder, Colorado. "It's a little like Toys 'R' Us: who can grab the attention first."

With dozens and dozens of tea boxes on the shelf, it's difficult to select a brand with the taste you prefer, especially when you can't see the tea leaves through the packaging. While there are more than 3,000 different varieties of teas, they are based mostly on the same four styles of tea—black, green, white, and oolong—each characterized by a different processing method. The only requirement on the package is tea; the rest of the wording is voluntary, so here are a few pointers to narrow down your favorite tea brand.

Tea Labeling

BLACK TEA

An American friend of mine, living in the U.K., quantifies her tea time by whether it's a tea bag moment or whether there is time for a pot of tea. Most Americans drink bag tea, black, with perhaps some sugar and lemon. When time allows, my preference is loose tea in a ceramic pot with warm milk, which lowers the tea's astringency and smoothes out the flavor.

Perhaps the most common term on boxes of American tea bags is "orange pekoe" (pronounced PĒ-kō). The term has nothing to do with orange-flavored tea or even a type of tea; rather, it's a leaf grade. To be called orange pekoe, the leaves must be handpicked from solely the youngest flower bud and the next two leaves.

Tea grading isn't standardized; each country has its own way of doing things. Some countries use an orthodox method, where the leaves are hand plucked and rolled. A new, more cost-efficient method for hand- or machine picking is CTC: Crush, Tear, and Curl.

Tea packaging will often emphasize that the tea is made with the tips plucked from the bud and the top three leaves. "With" is the key word; if the tea is made only from leaf tips it will say so. But "with" generally implies a blend of cut or crushed lower leaves and plucked top leaves.

Here are two examples of tea ingredient labels to test your tea leaf reading skills:

Assam, orange pekoe and cut pekoe: The tea is from Assam, a district in northeast India; orange pekoe is the top bud and two leaves of the tea plant, and cut pekoe is lower-grade pekoe made from cut leaves rather than whole leaves.

SFTGFOP1: This is a bit tougher. Tea graders also use letters and numbers as codes to judge teas. For instance, this is a Super Fine, Tippy Golden Flowery, Orange Pekoe grade 1 tea—or a mighty fine tea.

Assam, Darjeeling, Keemun, and So On   Teas are named after the regions where they are grown, similar to appellations in the wine industry. The most well-known are Assam, Darjeeling, Ceylon, Keemun, and Yunnan. Specialty teas may also include the name of the district or the garden (tea plantation). Here are a few taste descriptions of what to expect from assorted regions:

ASSAM (INDIA): Assam teas are good morning teas because they grab your attention with strong malt flavors. Assam teas are best with a bit of milk.

DARJEELING (INDIA): Darjeeling tea is grown along the foothills of the Himalayas and is known for its rarity and prestige. Spring-harvested

Darjeeling teas are soft and flowery; summer Darjeeling is darker and bolder. The English prefer Darjeeling for afternoon tea.

CEYLON (SRI LANKA): Ceylon tea is known for its astringent, liquorlike flavor and amber color. Ceylon teas are characterized by whether the leaves are grown at high, medium, or low elevations; high Ceylon is the best quality.

KEEMUN (CHINA): China's first-ever black tea has a subtle honey taste and flowery aroma.

YUNNAN (CHINA): Yunnan tea grows in the mountains bordering Vietnam, Laos, and Burma, China's largest tea-growing region. It's a full-tasting tea with a mochalike quality.

LAPSANG SOUCHONG (CHINA): Lapsang Souchong tea is made by withering tea leaves held over pine or cypress wood fires; hence the flavor is smoky, a little like a single-malt Scotch.

English, Scottish, and Irish Breakfast Tea Each of these teas was developed centuries ago in the British Isles to satisfy the tea taste buds of the English, Scottish, and Irish and offer a consistent tea blend in between harvesting seasons. While the blends vary among brands, English breakfast is a blend of teas like Ceylon, Assam, Nilgiri, and Keemun; Scottish tea is mostly Assam with some Kenyan. In Ireland, one of the world's biggest per capita tea-drinking countries, people like their *cuppan tae* the strongest of the lot, with Ceylon and Assam and a good splash of Irish milk. The Irish say their tea should be "strong enough for a mouse to trot on."

GREEN TEA

In 2005, the FDA nixed a petition for a qualified health claim, which cited green tea as a possible risk reducer for cancer, specifically breast and prostate. The snub didn't dampen the zeal of green tea lovers or even Sin Hang Lee, M.D., the man behind the claim, who said in a press release that he is "pleased that FDA is taking a look at this important issue."

The important issue is ever-increasing research that shows both black tea and green tea contain polyphenols known for cardiovascular health and enzymes that fight off cancer cell growth. The medical jury is still out on all the specific mechanics, but green tea has a strong connection to prevention of internal organ and skin cancer. The theory is that epigallocatechin-3-gallate (EGCG) prevents cancer cells from growing by binding to a specific enzyme that is the same target for cancer drugs. Green tea contains five times as much EGCG as black tea, but researchers estimate that even so, it may take more than five cups of green tea per day to see the optimum benefits.

Green tea is made from the same tea leaves as black tea, but some of the fresh qualities are preserved by steaming the leaves to inactivate the enzymes, which leaves a grassy flavor and bright green color. Chinese green tea is pan fried, giving it a roasted flavor and green-golden hue. India makes green tea as well, but in limited quantities. Chinese and Japanese green tea names are often a reflection of the shape of the leaves, such as gunpowder, pine needle, jade pillar, and pinhead.

WHITE TEA

White tea is considered one of the rarest teas, with the most delicate of flavors. The tea is made from the very top bud, whose delicate silvery threads make it look white. Researchers looking into this gem are noting that white tea has three times the level of antioxidants as green tea and standard black teas.

OOLONG TEA

Oolong tea, a cross between black and green tea, is considered the champagne of teas. The tea leaves are withered, then bruised and allowed to sit until the edges turn red. As with Chinese green tea, oolong is pan fried at a high temperature, rolled, and dried gently. The lengthy process crafts a fruity tea that needs no embellishments, such as milk, sugar, or lemon.

The most potent and interesting oolong is Pu-erh, named after a town in the Yunnan province of China. The ancient tea plant from which the leaves are picked is believed to hold restorative properties that help with indigestion, hangovers, cholesterol, and weight loss. Moreover, the tea has a funky shape and earthy taste. The large leaves are fermented twice for flavor and then shaped into tiny bowls that resemble birds' nests (*tuo chas*) and individually wrapped.

FLAVORED BLACK, GREEN, WHITE, AND OOLONG TEAS

The most widely known flavored tea is Earl Grey, perfumed with bergamot, a citrus fruit grown exclusively on the coast of Reggio Calabria, a province in southern Italy. According to legend, the tea was named after the Englishman Charles Earl Grey who, when on a diplomatic mission to China in 1803, was presented by a Chinese mandarin with the recipe for making this tea. Earl Grey tea leaves are generally a blend of Chinese black, Sri Lankan Ceylon, or Indian Darjeeling.

Black, green, white, and oolong teas are often scented with flowers such as jasmine, orchid, rose, and gardenia or combined with bits of dried fruit and pits such as mango, passion fruit, and peach. The practice is as much for flavor as it is to neutralize bitterness. Sunflower, calendula, and cornflower are particularly good at ridding tea of harsh tannins.

HERBAL TEA

If you want to raise the ire of a tea lover, call an herbal tea "tea." In reality, tea is a specific plant and that name is therefore reserved only for tea—not a blend of herbs, flowers, and fruit. The proper linguistic term for a steeped beverage other than tea is "herbal infusion" or "tisane."

The most well-known herbal infusion company in the United States is Celestial Seasonings, located a few miles from my front door in Boulder, Colorado. Mo Siegel founded the company by picking wild herbs in the forests and gorges near Aspen and Boulder. With the assistance of friends, he foraged enough wild stuff to package into hand-sewn muslin bags and sold them to a local health-food store. A few years later, the success of Red Zinger Herb Tea launched a homespun barn tea shop and the flower-picking entrepreneur, a manly one at that, into one of the most successful business ventures in the West.

Companies like Celestial Seasonings moved herbal blends from the medicinal category into beverages. Most herbal teas lack enough potent ingredients to serve as more than a soothing hot mug or a refreshing cold beverage. There are, however, a few companies that market their infusions as over-the-counter pharmaceuticals.

Medicinal teas are fine for non-life-threatening discomforts such as indigestion, constipation, minor cold relief, insomnia, and fatigue. For medicinal purposes look for pharmaceutical-grade teas. The formulations are based on European pharmacopoeias, which are monographs that outline the safe usage of herbal medicines. Read the usage information inside the box for side effects and contraindications, just as you would for an over-the-counter medicine. Herbs have medicinal properties that may interact with prescription drugs or exacerbate chronic conditions.

FAIR TRADE

Unlike coffee, in an industry dominated by small farms, tea is grown primarily on large plantations called gardens. Since tea must be processed within a very short time after harvest, the gardens are adjacent to the processing factories, which are simple rooms with wooden drying racks and screens for sifting and measuring the leaves. British colonial rule established a well-run system for tea, and jobs within the tea gardens are highly sought after. The conditions vary by region, but generally families live on the gardens in housing provided by the plantation owners, health care is provided, and children attend local schools.

All was relatively peaceful in tea town until recent years, when tea prices and demand fell. Jobs were cut and violence erupted among workers and plantation management; at least seven plantation bosses were lynched in 2004 in the state of Assam. Bengal also reported riots and killings among two Marxist government-affiliated trade unions fighting over the hiring of a tea office secretary.

A report by Action Aid, a nonprofit labor policy group in the U.K., shows that the tea industry is just beginning to see the same ill-fated symptoms as the coffee industry—demand for low-quality tea is declining, tea plantations need upgrading, and overabundant supplies are flooding the market.

Layoffs among tea pluckers are becoming more regular, and those lucky enough to keep their jobs are paid less for double the hours. The

Indian tea industry has taken a cue from the flourishing Indian computer help desk sector and begun outsourcing for contract labor to replace permanent tea workers. Tea pluckers are extraordinarily dependent on the remote plantations for housing, food, health care, and wages—laid-off workers have virtually nowhere to go for work.

Action Aid is calling for tea companies like Unilever (Lipton, Red Label, and PG Tips brands) to follow the lead of the coffee industry and support fair trade practices. The fair trade tea industry looks different from the coffee industry because it merges larger independent gardens with small farms into one co-op. Rodney North from Equal Exchange says the relationship is ideal, since the more experienced plantation growers can offer advice and support to the smaller-scale operation. To date there are a few fair trade tea lines available from Choice Teas, Stash, Equal Exchange, and Harney & Sons.

So while retail tea prices remain steady and shareholder dividends increase, wholesale auction tea prices are falling. Tea sales aren't based on a futures market, like coffee, so the assumption is that supply will generally match demand. Not so; tea auction houses are out of tune with buyer demand, and questionable practices among brokers and buyers are on the rise. All of these factors are leading tea down the same broken path as coffee. Action Aid is calling for Unilever (specifically the PG Tips tea brand) to apply fair trade practices to its tea suppliers, as well as influence other U.K.-based tea companies to follow suit.

Bottom Line

In July 2005, New York Exchange coffee prices appeared to be consistently above one dollar per pound for Arabica beans, owing to lower supplies and decreased acreage. Whether the farmer will pocket these gains is an unknown. And no one can predict whether the market will ever right itself permanently, which is why fair trade, ethical specialty coffee buyers, and grassroots entrepreneurial efforts play a collective role. There is more than enough room in the marketplace for all, especially when the benefit of paying a bit more for our morning java slows the rush of immigrants slipping across our border.

Tea is not only the world's most popular drink behind water, but it may also hold the Asian secrets to longevity and good health. Even coffee gets positive marks from the medical community. If we look beyond the limits of our own plush lives, both beverages hold up world economies and, more important, the lives of millions of farmers and workers living on the edge of survival and ruin. If you are one who frequently wakes in the morning, saying, "I can't live without my morning coffee" or "tea," remember there are millions of others who literally can't live without it.

CHAPTER 12

Crumbs and Crackers

America's Obsession with Sweet and Salty Snacks

While riding in an open jeep flanked by armed guards, his hired protectors in the Colombian jungle, every instinct must have told him otherwise, but Neil Blomquist is a man in the right place at the right time. The FDA's requirement for mandatory labeling of trans fats in 2006 turned this shy former CEO of Spectrum Naturals, a culinary oil company, into a twenty-first-century Indiana Jones.

Over an Oregon pinot noir at an Omaha restaurant, Blomquist shows me snapshots from his latest venture to the Colombian palm groves. This particular palm oil supplier strives to leave the smallest human footprint possible in the politically and environmentally sensitive rain forest. Instead of harvesting the fruit with heavy machinery, nimble men shimmy up palm trees with machetes, cutting away at the fruit by hand. Within earshot, voice-trained oxen stand by ready to haul wooden wagons brimming with fruit clusters to the nearby mill.

Spectrum has been a supplier of the trans fat–free tropical oil since the early 1980s—long before the FDA agreed that partially hydrogenated fats posed a health risk, and when few knew much about the slimy stuff. Now snack foods companies are looking to experts like Blomquist for fats that don't contain the heart-damaging components of trans fats and can keep up with the demand to satisfy Americans' love of sweet and salty, baked and fried snacks.

The 1980s marked the beginning of many new fads, including a misguided love for parachute pants and a vilification of all fats. Our fear was fueled by years of campaigns by food associations and citizens' and medical health groups against the use of saturated fats, such as lard, butter, and tropical oils, including palm and coconut.

Americans listened and threw out their grandmothers' lard piecrust recipes, margarine replaced butter, and "low-fat" cookies made with partially hydrogenated fats sold like hotcakes. Tropical fats were banished to their native island populations. Unfortunately, the increased use of partially hydrogenated fats—less saturated and more commercially stable fats than lard or butter—led us down a slick slope of ill health.

We should have defamed parachute pants instead; the misunderstanding about fats turned out to be a deadly mistake. Researchers now know that at least 30,000 people die each year of premature coronary heart disease as a result of eating partially hydrogenated fats from grocery store–bought food. The rate of heart disease jumps significantly higher when restaurant food is added to the equation. For each 2% increase in calories from partially hydrogenated fats, a woman's coronary risk escalates by 93%. Studies show that younger women's cardiovascular health is particularly affected by trans fats, another name for partially hydrogenated fats.

Phat Changes in Fats

Partially hydrogenated fats are made by bombarding unsaturated liquid vegetable oils, such as soybean, canola, cottonseed, and corn oil, with hydrogen gas and a metal catalyst (nickel or platinum). The process turns liquid fats into solids, which were once believed to be a solution to every commercial food processor's plight, including viscosity, flakiness, shelf life, and even reduced saturated-fat levels.

As the list of pros for partially hydrogenated fats grew within the food-manufacturing world, so did the list of cons from medical experts. The problem is that the shape and chemical structure of these fats are confusing to the human body, specifically tied to the way fats are metabolized. Fat molecules from liquid oils have fewer hydrogen bonds than saturated fats, allowing them to bend. These kinks help keep cells pliable and porous, which is good for our health. Saturated fats from, say, butter or lard pack together tightly, forming a straight molecule that the body recognizes and metabolizes appropriately when eaten sparingly—or stores as fat if eaten too often.

To transform a liquid fat into a solid partially hydrogenated fat, manufacturers add hydrogen molecules to some, but not all, of the available hydrogen bonds—hence the name partially hydrogenated. The resulting particles straighten out, forming a stiff molecule that looks to the human body a little like a saturated fat and a little like an unsaturated fat. Our bodies aren't programmed to recognize this fat, resulting in a cycle of metabolic bafflement.

Ultimately, the body tries and tries unsuccessfully to use partially hydrogenated fats as it would a liquid or a saturated fat. The fat has nowhere to go, so it builds up within the cardiovascular system and packs in around our organs, eventually leading to a host of diseases, including type 2 diabetes, insulin resistance, gallstones, degenerative arthritis, and cardiovascular disease.

You may think you are a careful shopper and have avoided partially hydrogenated fats at all costs, but it's doubtful that you dodged them all. Now that labeling is mandatory, they are easier to spot. However, unless you shop exclusively at a health-food store, where they are banned, use is pervasive. Prior to the labeling change, hydrogenated fats were in 154,000 brands or 307,600 individual products.

It's too soon to tell how many companies have switched to other fats. Depending on the number of products offered by a company, the labeling requirements for hydrogenated fats will cost each small food business an average of $9,300 to $18,000 to reformulate and/or label their brands. That's a drop in the bucket compared to the $900 million to $1.8 billion yearly savings in medical costs, lost productivity, and pain and suffering from illnesses caused by trans fats.

The transition away from hydrogenated fats means manufacturers have to find equally stable fats that are inexpensive and abundant. The options include new high-oleic canola and soy seed oils, fully hydrogenated vegetable oil, and tropical fats. The healthiest of these choices are liquid oils, though as any good baker knows, cookies need a little solid fat for texture and taste, which is where fully hydrogenated oils and tropical fats come into play.

The bad science that pushed tropical fats aside is being overshadowed by positive research about fully hydrogenated fats, coconut and palm fruit oil. Researchers suspect that although these fats are saturated and should be eaten in moderation, they are cholesterol neutral, meaning they have no negative impact on cholesterol levels. Though the "too much of anything" rule still applies with tropical oils, a small amount every now and again may not be as bad as was once believed.

Now that scientists are reanalyzing the science, there is a growing understanding that palm and coconut oils raise good cholesterol levels and do not influence the heart-damaging types. The phenomenon may be from a fatty acid called lauric acid, which is very abundant in coconut oil and less so in palm. Lauric acid raises healthy cholesterol levels more than any other fatty acid—saturated or not.

With this knowledge, food manufacturers are turning toward palm and coconut oils for their new product formulations. When reading labels, look for palm fruit oil, which is 50% saturated, as compared to palm kernel at 86% saturation. Coconut oil is 92% saturated, but again it contains lauric acids, known for raising healthy cholesterol, as well as antiviral and antibacterial properties.

After years of being on the fringe, health-food companies are being courted by mainstream food manufacturers for their knowledge of liquid vegetable oils and coconut and palm fruit oil as acceptable alternatives to partially hydrogenated fats. The cycle has come full circle, putting Blomquist and companies like his in the right place, at just the right time.

Dissecting Snack Labels

It's not an oxymoron: Health and snack foods can share the same table and the same sentence. Healthy snack foods are one of the top-selling food categories. There are, however, imposters, which can be flushed out with some careful label reading. Here are some healthy and not so healthy labels to look for.

OLESTRA

I'm not sure that any other new food product introduction has made broadcast journalists squirm as much as this one. A seemingly innocuous story about potato chips introduced consumers to not only a new food but also the term "anal leakage"—not an easy phrase for even the most professional news anchor to say with a straight face on national television.

The clamor and squirming was over Procter & Gamble's Olestra, an oil-like compound with molecules so large they pass right through our digestive tract without being absorbed. Product developers at P&G were hopeful that Olestra would be used in hundreds of full-fat products, such as baked goods and snack foods, transforming them from forbidden fruit into guilt-free foods.

No matter how good it sounded, there was one side effect that couldn't be ignored by the media, consumer groups, physicians, and the FDA—anal leakage. Since the fat essentially slides through the digestive tract, it can cause gastrointestinal discomfort and take some of the fat-soluble nutrients vitamins A, D, E, and K with it.

P&G sponsored numerous scientific and consumer sampling studies to overcome the negative image. The aggressive pursuit for approval from the FDA and the medical community drew criticisms because most of the positive studies regarding Olestra came from P&G-sponsored research. Some saw the oil as a solution to the obesity crisis; others noted that even fat-free potato chips were still empty calories and that the oil might cause vitamin depletions.

After a decade of wrangling, in 1996 the FDA approved use of the oil in salty snack foods, sold under Frito-Lay's WOW! brand, as long as a warning label stated the following:

This product contains Olestra. Olestra may cause abdominal cramping and loose stools. Olestra inhibits the absorption of some vitamins and other nutrients. Vitamins A, D, E, and K have been added.

In 2003, the FDA removed the warning label, agreeing that there were adequate postapproval studies showing Olestra causes no more gastric discomfort than a high-fiber diet, rich in fruits and whole grains. In 2004, Frito-Lay announced that Olestra-made chips would switch from the brand name WOW! to "Light." Two years later, a thirty-seven-year-old woman was hospitalized with severe abdominal pain, vomiting, and diarrhea after eating Olestra-fried chips. To prevent a lawsuit, Frito-Lay agreed to change the packaging to include an Olean logo (the fat brand) on the front panel, as well as a banner that says "made with Olestra."

The underpinnings of Olestra's approval process are best described in Marion Nestle's book, *Food Politics: How the Food Industry Influences Nutrition and Health* (University of California Press, 2003). Nestle devotes an entire chapter to the chronology and conflicts regarding the Olestra approval process. I recommend the book for a close-up look at the issues regarding the politics of ingredient approvals and food labeling.

TRANS FATS OR PARTIALLY HYDROGENATED FATS

The very same company that took the chance in launching Olestra-fried chips was the first to begin reformulating their products by completely removing partially hydrogenated fats from some brands of Fritos and Lays potato chips. Frito-Lay has been in the forefront of oil research, by switching to a new sunflower oil, NuSun, that is low in saturated fat, with no trans fats, but is stable enough for food production. When liquid oils are deodorized during extraction, the process creates tiny amounts of trans fats, which are not that significant to health, though the NuSun oil has no consequential trans fats.

Other companies, such as Pepperidge Farm (Goldfish) and Nabisco (TRISCUIT crackers), have also reformulated their products. As of this writing not all brands within these companies have removed all the trans fats, so read the entire ingredient label carefully.

Even with the label change, there is still an ambiguity allowing manufacturers to say their products are trans fat free, though it's not entirely true. A labeling leniency allows marketers to say a product has 0g of trans fats if there is less than .5g per serving. FDA is considering lowering the level to .2g.

If you eat more than a single serving of snack foods, and who doesn't, you may easily exceed the .5g acceptable limit. The FDA made the decision for two reasons: (1) It's difficult to accurately test for trans fats in levels below .5g, and (2) the agency believes that since it's impossible to totally eliminate all trans fats from one's diet, a half of a gram of trans fats poses a negligible risk. The Institute of Medicine (IOM), the group that determines the recommended dietary allowances for nutrients, disagrees, noting that any level of trans fats is unhealthy.

With the .5g rule, it's not enough to only read the nutritional panel; read all the ingredients. For instance, a product may say "0 grams trans fats, per serving," or "trans-fat free, per serving," but still list partially hydrogenated vegetable oils in the ingredients. The "per serving" clause should raise a mental red flag. For a truly trans fat–free snack food, look for labels that say "contains no trans fats," but still check the ingredient list.

NATURAL

Although the term "natural" doesn't have any clout in the food-labeling kingdom, it implies the snack food ingredients, such as flavorings and preservatives, are not synthetic and there is minimal processing. "Minimal processing" is a loose term, especially for processed foods. Corn syrup is one example; in conventional stores corn syrup is considered a natural product, while health-food stores forbid the sticky stuff.

Since there aren't any controls to define the term "natural," "organic" is the only guarantee that the chips or cookies are made from nonsynthetic sources such as dairy cultures for cheese flavorings and citric acid and fruit for sweet flavors, as compared to artificial flavorings and colors used in conventional products. If a manufacturer can't find an organic flavoring ingredient, they may use a conventional approved ingredient, provided it doesn't represent more than 5% of the product.

REDUCED FAT

Reduced-fat products contain 25% less fat than a full-fat counterpart product. This does not mean that the fat remaining in the product will be any healthier for you. For instance, one brand of cookies popular among weight-conscious shoppers says "reduced fat"; however, the ingredients list partially hydrogenated soybean oil as the primary fat source. So while you may be eating 3g less fat than the regular version, you are still getting a whopping 5g of trans fats—the worst possible type. Again, it's as much about the type of fats as the quantity.

Salty chip companies have been more successful with reduced-fat product formulations than baked-good manufacturers. The process is proprietary; however, reduced-fat kettle-fried chips seem to offer the lowest saturated fat levels at .5g. The end product has fewer calories, 40% less fat, and no trans fats. According to my own family's taste test, there is little or no taste difference from the higher-fat varieties. Baked chips are also low in fat, although for some brands the flavored coatings may contain small amounts of partially hydrogenated fats.

If you still want your cake, cookies, or chips (and to eat them, too) look for products made with all or mostly liquid vegetable oils, preferably with more monounsaturated fats and less polyunsaturated; any high-oleic oil qualifies (such as NuSun or canola). For baked goods, the advice is the same, although the ingredients will most likely also include some solid fats—look for small amounts of coconut and palm fruit oil, fully hydrogenated vegetable oils, and, if your diet allows, a tad of old-fashioned butter.

REDUCED SUGAR/SUGAR FREE

For insulin-sensitive and diabetic consumers, this marketing message may be outwardly attractive, until you read the nutrition label. When product formulators take out sugar, they have to replace it with something else to maintain the original taste and texture—usually fats, sugar alcohols, and other types of carbohydrates. It's a case of robbing Peter to pay Paul, which is never a good solution.

Depending on what is added, the final product may have less granulated sugar but overall isn't any healthier than the original formulation. For instance, when sugar is replaced with refined carbohydrates like maltodextrin (made from corn starch), the product still holds the same number of calories and overall carbohydrates as the original version.

Sugar alcohols, made from manipulated sugars from fruits, trees, and other plants, are a common way to take out the sugar in commercial baked goods. With half the sweetness and calories of sugar, they are absorbed more slowly into the bloodstream and therefore have less impact on glucose levels.

Sugar alcohols aren't entirely free of calories, though. Dieticians say if you eat large amounts of sugar alcohols, they can affect blood sugar levels and cause embarrassing gastric problems. Five grams or less per serving has a minimal effect.

When a product uses only one type of sugar alcohol, the ingredients panel will list the individual name. The collective term "sugar alcohols" mean more than one type is used. Common terms are "sorbitol," "lactitol," "xylitol," "mannitol," "maltitol," "erythritol," "dulcitol," "starch hydrolysates," and "isomalt."

If a product says "sugar-free," and this issue is important to your health, make certain that the fats are healthy and the total calories, carbohydrates, and sugar alcohols are not excessive. Here's how too many sugar alcohols can add up: Sugar has four calories per gram; sugar alcohols have two calories per gram. So if a serving size contains 24g of sugar alcohols, that is the calorie equivalent of 12g of regular sugar, or four to five teaspoons—hardly a sugar-free product. Again, try to stay within the 5g-per-serving limit.

HIGH PROTEIN

Americans love to nosh on healthy and not so healthy snacks. As food formulators figure out how to improve the health profile, you will see more new products touting the benefits of high-protein and low-fat snack foods, especially meal replacement bars.

They look like candy bars, but don't misunderstand: Energy bars are intended for use as meal replacements. Product developers pack the bars with soy and whey protein to satisfy the needs of über-athletes, people who need quick and lasting energy because of rigorous training schedules. For the rest of us, who are lucky to get in a thirty-minute walk, the dense calories can lead to weight gain, especially if eaten too frequently. In addition, some of these bars contain high levels of soy protein and as much as the 100% RDA for vitamins.

If you take vitamin pills and eat other soy products, collectively the levels of some nutrients may be too high.

Corn and soy chips are another high-protein snack source. The protein comes from soybean grits, soy flour, sesame seeds; hemp, and bean flakes. These products tout low-carb and protein-rich ingredients that are a bit healthier than other snack foods, but the calories can add up, so don't munch with complete abandon.

There are three types of protein claims: high protein—10g or more of high-quality protein per serving; good source of protein—at least 5g of high-quality protein per serving; and more protein—at least 5g more of high-quality protein per serving than reference food.

If a single serving is low in total and saturated fat and low in cholesterol and contains as much as 6.25g of soy protein, a meal replacement bar or snack food can carry a soy health claim. The claim states: *"Diets low in saturated fat and cholesterol that include 25 grams of soy protein a day may reduce the risk of heart disease."*

WHOLE GRAIN

Few of us get the recommended 48g of whole grains in our diet, and despite the marketing terms "added whole grain" and "made with whole grains," you won't get enough from crackers carrying these terms. Perhaps they are an attempt to relieve our guilt, but most of the snack products that say "with" or "added whole grains" only have 1 or 2g of fiber, which is a long way from 48g. In addition, these products may also contain partially hydrogenated fats, making the benefits of a trivial amount of fiber null and void.

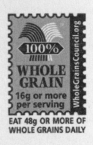

To find products that contain more than a token amount of whole grains, look for this stamp. The Whole Grains Council (a food association of grain millers, food scientists, and chefs affiliated with a food think tank called Oldways) has come up with this label to draw attention to whole-grain products. The label will note the number of grams of whole grain in a single serving, with a reminder that we all need 48g or more of whole grains per day.

NET CARBS AND LOW CARBS

Until the FDA agrees on the meaning of "net carbs" and "low carbs," there is a lot of wiggle room with this label. The label was conjured up by manufacturers to attract low-carb food followers, and the interpretation varies significantly. In the snack category, some products, such as nuts, naturally meet the low-carb concept; others need some reformulation, usually by adding fiber and taking out some sugar.

The term "net carbs" is based on the concept that higher fibrous carbohydrates are digested more slowly than refined carbohydrates, resulting in lower blood sugar levels. Manufacturers come up with this net-carb number by subtracting the grams of fibrous carbohydrates and grams of sugar alcohols from the total number of carbohydrates. While adding more fiber and taking out some sugar from your diet isn't a bad change for snack foods, the definition of "low carb" differs from one company to another. If you follow a low-carb diet, instead of relying on marketing terms read the label for the type of carbohydrates, such as whole grains and low sugars—your definition of "low carb" may not match that of the manufacturer (see the grains chapter for more on low carbs and glycemic index).

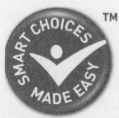

TM SNACK HEALTHY

The big three names in snack foods have recently adopted labels to help consumers identify healthier choices. The labels Sensible Snacking, Smart Spot, and Choices, used by Kraft Foods (the company declined reproduction of the seal in this book), PepsiCo, and Unilever (no graphic available), respectively, are approved for snack foods that have calorie, sugar, sodium, and fat restrictions.

The Pepsi Smart Spot label has similar criteria. Products contain at least 10% of the DV of a targeted nutrient (i.e., protein, fiber, calcium, iron, vitamin A, vitamin C) and meet limits for fat, saturated fat, trans fat, cholesterol, sodium, and added sugar, or they are formulated to have specific health or wellness benefits, or they have reduced calories or nutrients such as fat, sodium, or sugar.

The "Sensible Snacking" seal was developed by Kraft's nutrition experts, and the nutrition criteria are derived from the 2005 U.S. Dietary Guidelines, authoritative statements from the FDA, and input by a health and wellness advisory council. The criteria for each food will be reviewed every six months. The foods provide nutrients such as protein, calcium, or fiber/whole grain at nutritionally meaningful levels or deliver a functional benefit, such as heart health or hydration, while staying within specific limits on calories, fat (including saturated and trans fat), sodium, and sugar or by meeting specifications for "reduced," "low," or "free" in calories, fat, saturated fat, sugar, or sodium.

The labels are a smart move that helps with portion control and calories. The only fault I find with the products is that some still contain low levels of trans fats and sugar, which I hope will be phased out in time.

THE OREO DEBATE

I'm not alone when I say that Oreos are one of my favorite junk foods. Since the early 1900s billions of people have adored this coveted snack. Whether you twist and scrape out the creamy center or dunk the cookie intact into a glass of cold milk, it's pure bliss. I practice what I preach. So about a decade ago, when the warnings about trans fats first trickled out, I gave Oreos up cold turkey. Now I indulge in a few similar cookies on my birthday, but the brand is Nell and Paul Newman's trans fat–free sandwich cookie.

Given my appreciation for the cookie, it's natural that this chapter include a bit of history about the lawsuit that crumbled Kraft's reliance on partially hydrogenated fats for Oreo cookies. Stephen L. Joseph, founder, president, and legal representative for BanTransFats.com, Inc., a consumer advocacy group, sued Kraft Foods on May 1, 2003. The suit was based on a California product liability law (California Civil Code Section 1714.45), which states that a manufacturer or seller can be held liable if the dangers of a food product are not adequately disclosed to the average consumer.

In this case, the product was Oreos, the consumers were Californians, specifically children, and the liability was that consumers (children and their parents) didn't have fair warning regarding the amount of partially hydrogenated fats in the creamy center, even though there was an Oreo food marketing campaign in schools. By May 3, the suit caught the attention of every major media outlet in the world.

Critics accused Joseph of pandering to the media with the frivolous lawsuit. Joseph says he simply asked for an injunction ordering Kraft, after a reasonable grace period, to cease and desist from marketing and selling Oreo cookies to children in the state of California until the cookies contained no partially hydrogenated oil.

At this point the suit was no longer valid, says Joseph, since everyone who wanted to know now knew about trans fats. "The suit was a victim of its own success," he says. Just one day after filing the suit, there was enough awareness to prompt Kraft to agree to get the trans fats out of Reduced Fat Oreo, Golden Oreo Originals, and Golden Uh Oh! Oreo brands. (Now even the regular brand is trans fat–free).

Joseph's timing of the lawsuit was questioned by legal ethics pundits, since the suit was presented days before the FDA announced the mandatory trans fats labeling rule. Despite what you may think of Joseph's litigious tactics, this author thinks his motives were well founded. I also commend Kraft for moving quickly to remove the partially hydrogenated fats from a few brands. Joseph's actions fast-forwarded awareness of the issue to light-speed proportions, since the FDA ruling was three years away from being mandatory.

Even parents who weren't likely to read a dry, buried newspaper story about FDA food labeling laws now knew about the risks of trans fats—long before the damage was done to their children's health. Unfortunately for Kraft, which was not the only trans fat culprit in the food world, it became the vehicle for this particular message.

Joseph will tell you this was not a case about money; it was about marketing junk food directly to children, who have no way of understanding the dangers of partially hydrogenated fats. The suit pointed

(continued)

out that although parents are still the ultimate guardians of their children's eating habits, the lack of trans fat quantities on the ingredient panel prevented parents from making wise decisions. Moreover, the parents didn't have control over an Oreo school-marketing campaign called "Oreo Online Project," reaching 12,000 children in forty-three states and overseas.

So why did Joseph choose Oreos and Kraft? Although he might have liked to, he couldn't sue everyone. The popular cookie was a highly visible target, representing one of the most successful brands in packaged food history. In fact, he initially disagreed with me about putting his story about trans fats in this particular chapter. "By putting this in the snack foods chapter, you will give the impression that trans fats are only in junk food," he said. "It makes some think that the people who eat this type of food deserve what they get. It's in every type of food in the store."

He's right; trans fats are in every type of food, including cookies, seemingly healthy cereals, puddings, pastries, coffee creamer, margarines, and even some beverages. Since book space is limited, I chose to put trans fats here. However, take Joseph's advice; don't ignore the other smaller references to trans fats in almost every chapter of this book—no one is any less important than the other.

Last, he says, remember that the trans fat problem isn't limited to the grocery stores; restaurants have become equally reliant on the fat. During the same week as our conversation, McDonald's began test marketing a new trans fat–free frying oil and posting warning signs on its California drive-through windows and doors about the health risks of trans fats. The warning signs may change the company's motto from "Billions Sold," to "Billions Told."

CHAPTER 13

Aisle of Denial:
Carbonated and Sweetened Beverages

Kicking the Soda Can Habit

Friends question my sanity, but one of my favorite classes involves teaching high school teens to cook. In between lessons in knife skills and sautéing, I sneak in a few tips on healthy cooking and eating. It never fails that at least one student will come to class slurping a tall soda through a long straw—that's my cue to bring up the subject of sugary drinks.

I start with a visual, a plastic bag with a few inches of sugar. "How much sweetener is this?" The answers vary from a few teaspoons to a cup, but they always use common cooking measurements such as teaspoons, tablespoons, and cups—not grams, as is listed on soda cans.

"How many grams is this?" Silence. To these teens, luckily, the only people who talk about plastic bags and grams are chemistry teachers and drug pushers in the movies. My answer of "39g" gets another bored look. When I add, "This is nine and three-quarters teaspoons, the same amount in a twelve-ounce soda," even these hard-to-astound teens gasp.

"Now, how many soft drinks do you drink per day? Or do you prefer fountain drinks with bottomless refills?" It never fails that someone will shout out, "What about lemonade and iced tea?" To answer, I hold up the same bag. With raised eyebrows and guilty looks, the class mentally adds up the number of teaspoons of sweetener they consume every day. While I have their attention, we talk about food choices, balancing calories with physical activity, and then move on to something more fun—cooking.

Obesity is on the rise for teens and adults, and no doubt too many soft drinks are one of the reasons, along with eating too much and exercising too little. Sweet drinks have become the beverage of choice, increasing our calorie intake by 135% since 1977. Government data show that teen males drink about two soft drinks per day, females slightly less. A whopping 20% of teen males drink as many as five soft drinks per day; females, three. Equally concerning is that as intake of soft drinks goes up, milk consumption goes down, especially among children and teens, at a time when bone growth is crucial for old age— even though teens firmly believe they will never be as old as we are.

The additional calories are insidious, say obesity experts. A study at an after-school day-care center shows how easily the pounds can add up, even for active younger children. Children who drank more than sixteen ounces of sweet beverages per day for two months gained two and a half pounds, compared to weight gain of no more than one pound for those who drank six to sixteen ounces of sweetened drinks per day. If this pattern continued, these kids could put on an extra fifteen pounds per year, well beyond normal growth expectations.

Parents blame the schools and lawmakers blame the soft drink industry for tempting underfunded schools with much-needed revenue from vending machine sales. The soft drink industry blames the kids for lack of restraint and the parents for a lack of oversight. Physicians point to too many nutritionally void calories and no exercise. There is most likely more than one cause, but as the number of overweight children climbs well into double digits, the resulting health issues of early onset of diabetes and heart disease are an ominous predictor of the poor health of our nation overall.

The biggest hurdle to getting rid of soft drinks isn't the kids; it's the money. Attempts to ban soft drinks from schools altogether have been met by strong opposition because of the large revenue streams associated with vending machines—often reaching into hundreds of thousands of dollars for each school district. It's no secret that schools need revenue. Parents are asking: At whose expense?

One such parent and maverick of healthy eating, Gary Hirshberg, CEO of the Stonyfield Farm organic yogurt company, developed a healthy vending machine program that competes nickel for nickel

with major vendors, such as Coke and Pepsi. The program, called
Menu for Change, lets the students decide which healthy snacks and
beverages go into the machines with student-run marketing and taste-
testing campaigns. The Menu for Change vending machines don't replace other vendors; they sit alongside the standard mix of soft-drink
and junk-food machines. Much to the surprise of administrators,
profits have doubled in the twenty-six schools participating in the program. Other school districts that have eliminated sweet drinks and
junk food from vending machines also report a rise in profits or, at the
least, negligible changes. Perhaps it *is* the adults who are getting in
the students' way.

The argument for soda machines in schools is much like the tobacco industry's early attempts to pigeonhole smoking into a corner
of behavior called personal responsibility. This spin might work for
adult behavior, but since adults *are* responsible for protecting children
from all health risks from birth to the last vestiges of adolescence, the
argument hasn't gained much support.

The American Beverage Association (ABA) fended off some verbal
and legal blows by announcing a plan to limit the availability of soft
drinks in elementary and middle schools until the final bell. The true
indicator of whether the beverage industry was offering merely a token measure or a genuine response was high schools. The age group
that needed the most restraint got the least help. High school vending
machines would contain 50% sodas.

Soon after Connecticut considered banning the sale of soft drinks
in schools, the fourth state to do so, the ABA finally agreed to voluntarily remove all sweetened drinks from elementary and middle
school vending machines by 2009. In place of sweetened drinks, the
machines will contain water, milk, and juice. High school machines
still had fewer restrictions, allowing for sports drinks, diet sodas, and
low-calorie juice drinks.

Brokers of the agreement, the William J. Clinton Foundation and
the American Heart Association, say the change came about from ne-
gotiations, not a threat of lawsuits. However, lawyers well versed in
the tobacco industry were waiting in the wings to see the outcome. It's
not over yet; the soft drink industry may have to jump from one frying

pan to the other—this time it's about the ingredients. The latest targets are high-fructose corn syrup and benzoate.

Is High-Fructose Corn Syrup the Next Food Villain?

I don't use the word "sugar" when I show the students how much sweetener is in a soft drink. I'm a stickler for detail, and depending on their attention span, I tell them the sweet stuff in soft drinks is mostly high-fructose corn syrup (HFCS), made from cornstarch. High sugar prices in the 1970s led food and beverage manufacturers to switch to cheaper HFCS, increasing consumption of HFCS by 1000%, from a mere half pound per person in 1970 to sixty-two pounds in 2003— mostly from beverages.

Is the parallel rise in HFCS usage and the diseases of obesity and diabetes linked? Or is it the abundance of food and lack of exercise? It may be a little of both. First and foremost, in the land of plenty Americans eat way more than we used to of all types of food, adding about 200 excess calories per day. With calories up and activity levels down, these factors alone are enough to cause steady weight gain and health problems.

It's not coincidental, say other researchers, that the sharp increase in certain health conditions mirrors the increase in HFCS tonnage in our food supply. If one compares sugar consumption alone from the seventies until now, it's declined per capita by almost thirteen pounds, while HFCS intake is now at sixty-two pounds. Combine this with a better understanding of the way we metabolize HFCS and the link gets stronger. High consumption of HFCS may aggravate an increasingly common syndrome called insulin resistance—a cluster of problems related to high blood pressure and high blood fats and cholesterol, which can lead to diabetes.

Here is what researchers believe thus far. When we eat or drink something sweet from foods with sugar (sucrose), the hormone insulin jumps in to help the body convert sugar to glucose—the body's primary energy source. When the body has all it needs, insulin triggers another hormone called leptin, a hormone that tells the brain to ebb appetite.

The emerging research suggests the insulin–leptin process might be sidestepped when high amounts of HFCS get into the bloodstream. Researchers suspect that a specific type of HFCS fructose, called free fructose, may be the culprit (HFCS in sweetened drinks contains 42 to 55% free fructose). While the mechanics aren't yet fully understood, researchers are fairly certain that free fructose can interfere with normal carbohydrate and fat metabolism and cause major metabolic changes, throwing off the body's normal reaction to blood sugars.

This excess blood sugar eventually gets stored as fat primarily in and around the liver and abdominal tissue. Fructose also increases levels of dangerous fat cells in our blood called triglycerides—markers of heart disease. "Fructose seems to be highly lipogenic, meaning it can turn into fat very quickly," says Dr. Khosrow Adeli, head and professor of clinical biochemistry at the Hospital for Sick Children, University of Toronto. "We noticed that problems tended to develop very quickly, much quicker than we expected, including higher body weight, high blood pressure, high lipid levels, and high cholesterol."

This connection is well understood in laboratory animals, like dogs, mice, and hamsters. For the human race, the association between unregulated blood sugar, obesity, and HFCS is gaining acceptance as new research emerges. Recent discoveries about a specific gene, called PTP-1B, show that individuals with an abundance of this genetic material are prone to problems with insulin resistance, which adds another layer of complexity, as well as clarity, to the matter. Interestingly, fructose ingestion has been recently shown to induce expression of the PTP-1B gene, which can in turn lead to the insulin resistance syndrome and diabetic complications, Adeli says.

It's only natural that the soft drink industry and Corn Refiners Association refute the studies' outcome. They cite the notion that no food is a bad food if consumed in moderation. Scientists don't dispute that and admit that the research is new, posing some doubt as to whether the weight of our problems is entirely a result of HFCS or it's genetic makeup, overindulgence, or a combination of all of these factors. Nevertheless, for our children's sake and our own, the advice to limit soft drink consumption doesn't really need any further research to back it up—does it?

Benzene

A lesser concern, but one that illustrates the inadequate self-regulation in the soft drink industry, is benzoate, an antimicrobial that when combined with ascorbic acid may create benzene, a carcinogen. The concerns about benzoate are not new. In the 1990s drink formulators came across the combination of ingredients, especially in orange- and other citrus-flavored soft drinks, that caused the formation of benzene. Soft drink makers promised the FDA that they could solve the problem by themselves, without government regulation.

By 2005, benzene again showed up in private laboratory tests, the levels high enough to warrant concern and a call for action. The FDA disagreed, saying there were no safety concerns but that an investigation was under way. The difference in opinion is likely due to differences in testing methods. The FDA tests for benzene may have been inadequate because the agency tested refrigerated drinks, not warm beverages. If the drinks are stored in high temperatures and exposed to light, such as stacked up in front of a gas station on a summer day or even in the backseat of a hot car, the benzene levels may well exceed the EPA's limits for drinking water. For some products, the private tests showed levels that were as high as 89 ppb—the EPA calls for public notification for drinking water at 5 ppb.

The benzene beverage snafu is a snapshot of self-regulation gone awry. A number of new beverage companies never got the memo regarding this potentially dangerous combination of ingredients, and even the well-established beverage companies lost some corporate knowledge over the last fifteen years. In addition, the FDA testing regulations had not been updated for plastic-bottled noncarbonated drinks.

FDA-sponsored tests showed private label brands as well as major brands containing ascorbic acid with excessive benzene levels. All of the brands with high benzene levels were fruit and citrus-flavored soft drinks, most often diet products.

Medical experts all commented that the high calories in soft drinks pose more of a risk to health than the occasional exposure to benzene—nonetheless, they say, it shouldn't be present in foods. Drink formulators have promised to once again reformulate their products. By the time you read this, the problem will most likely have been resolved—but just in case you find some long-forgotten plastic-bottled drinks stored away in a hot garage or in the storeroom at the high school sports concession stand, read the label. If you see benzoate and ascorbic acid or erythorbic acid and fruit juice (especially citrus or cherry), toss them out.

Beverage Labeling

SWEETENERS

To accommodate fluctuating formulations and sweetener prices, the soft drink industry has pushed for decades to allow "and/or" wording within the ingredient list, such as "sucrose and/or high-fructose corn syrup." In 2005, the FDA declared such labeling wasn't warranted— so beverage makers will have to list the exact ingredients in the future. If nothing else, remember one thing when shopping for drinks: Every 4g of sugars equals one teaspoon of sweetener, and every teaspoon is about fifteen calories. So, for instance, a twelve-ounce sweetened drink with 40g of sugars is ten teaspoons, or 150 calories.

SUGAR SUBSTITUTES

As a teen, I was oblivious to safety questions surrounding sugar substitutes—I remember downing my fair share of Tab colas after cheerleading and track practice. Today teens and adults have more than one brand of controversy to choose from. The number of consumers swapping sweetened drinks for diet drinks is so great that diet drink sales growth has surpassed the flatline statistics for sugared soft drink sales.

The first two sugar substitutes, *cyclamates* and *saccharine*, shared the same levels of scientific angst and political pressure for approval. Both were implicated in studies showing a potential risk for cancers in animals, not humans. The animal studies were enough to ban cyclamates in 1969. Saccharin survived the scrutiny, in part due to changes in the regulatory atmosphere a decade later.

The only admission of any problem was an FDA cancer warning label for saccharin, but it was rescinded in 2000 because of a lack of substantial evidence since saccharin's introduction into the food supply. Early research showed that mice were inclined to develop bladder cancer from copious amounts of saccharin-sweetened sodas. For humans there was a small connection with six servings or more per day, but according to regulators, this was not enough to require the warning label any longer. Here are the other sugar substitutes that have come along since then and the latest research regarding their safety.

Aspartame   Even after twenty-five years, aspartame is still a target for those who question its safety and cry collusion between the powerful parent company, Monsanto, and the FDA. Criticism comes from two ends of the spectrum—on one side are groups that compare aspartame to the evils of the Third Reich; on the other are medical experts who question the legitimacy of the science behind the approval process. Clearly, the Third Reich conspiracy theorists have bigger issues than only aspartame.

The concern among antiaspartame scientists is that it can create conditions within the brain that are ideal for brain tumors, cause disorders within the nervous system, and lead to autoimmune diseases. In April 2006, a federally sponsored study, one without any conflict of interest or industry funding, may have solved the argument once and for all. Scientists at the National Cancer Institute reviewed aspartame intake of more than 340,000 men and 225,000 women. Over a five-year period, the researchers could find no link between aspartame consumption and the blood and brain cancers that developed among the test subjects.

Just prior to the National Cancer Institute study, an Italian researcher released findings that the sweetener may be associated with high rates of lymphomas and leukemia in rats. The study fueled the long-held opinions of those who believe the sweetener should be removed from the market. So the argument continues. The only indisputable fact the Italian study may have confirmed is that it isn't wise for an adult to drink five 20-ounce diet sodas a day for seven years, as the rats were forced to do.

There is an indisputable warning regarding aspartame for people with phenylketonuria (PKU), a rare, inherited metabolic disease that can result in mental retardation and neurological problems without treatment. The disorder is because of a missing enzyme (phenylalanine hydroxylase), and aspartame contains 50% phenylalanine, which exacerbates the condition.

Splenda   For consumers who prefer to avoid aspartame, sucralose (brand name Splenda) is the newest sugar substitute in the beverage aisle. It's made by replacing three hydrogen and oxygen molecules in sugar with a chlorine molecule. Splenda's media campaign that it "tastes like sugar, because it's made from sugar" has fueled complaints from the sugar industry, citing unfair advertising practices.

The "made from sugar" claim has the health-food industry in a quandary and has led to a disagreement as to whether sucralose is "natural enough" to be allowed on store shelves or should be shunned. The debate opened the door for sugar alcohols to be marketed as "natural" as well, because they are derived from foods like milk, mushrooms, fruits, and vegetables. The sugar industry would like to see that only cane and beet sugar be deemed natural. Since the word "natural" lacks clarity in all food sectors, the argument remains unresolved.

With regard to serious health problems from sugar substitutes, any positive connections seem to be associated with animal studies using extreme amounts over extended periods of time. If you find that you are sensitive to any given product, there are plenty of options within the diet beverage market, or you can always simply stick with water—a truly natural beverage.

Sugar Alcohols   The latest addition to the "sugar-free" drink market is sugar alcohols. These sweet molecules made from plant and tree fibers cause a slow increase in blood sugar. They have anywhere from one-half to three-quarters the calories of regular sugar, so they are not entirely calorie free. They are, however, much sweeter than sugar, so manufacturers use much less than sugar. Their biggest drawback is intestinal distress, so go easy. Sugar alcohols are recognizable by the suffix "itol": lactitol, sorbitol, mannitol, xylitol.

PORTION SIZE

America's generous consumption of sweet drinks is as much about lack of restraint as increased portion sizes. When we hold a beverage bottle or can in our hand, mentally it's one serving, but in reality it may be as many as three servings. This is particularly true for large cans and bottles that cannot be resealed—our tendency is to finish it all.

Reading drink labels is an exercise in frustration. Just what is a single serving? Is it eight ounces, or is it twelve ounces? A sixteen-ounce bottle is listed as two servings, but the sugar content on the nutrition panel is for only one serving. The pressure is on for beverage manufacturers to draw attention to serving sizes and calories, as well as provide a double column of values for nutrients per serving and per package. Until then, you'll have to do the math yourself.

ENERGY DRINKS

The energy drink market is an explosive category filled with tiny cans and tall bottles promising to boost us out of our sleep-deprived daily ruts and inspire us to take up extreme sports like skydiving and glacier snowboarding. They do this with lots of caffeine, sweeteners, and a smattering of vitamins and medicinal herbs.

Don't be fooled—many of these drinks are extreme all right, extremely high in caffeine and sweeteners. Rather than use the "C" word, it's much cooler to use words like "guaranine" and "mateine," which refer to plant-derived sources of caffeine. No matter the language, these products contain anywhere from 50 to 400mg of caffeine per product—a jittery revelation in comparision to a shot of espresso with 40mg of caffeine. In addition, an eight-ounce serving can pack as much as nine teaspoons of sweetener. The large bottles are saturated with as much as twenty-two teaspoons.

The vitamins, minerals, and amino acids in energy drinks look like a chapter from a sports supplement how-to manual. The most common are taurine (regulates the heart muscle), B vitamins (for physical stress), carnitine (for fat metabolism), and creatine, a performance-enhancing supplement banned by the National Collegiate Athletic Association.

Ginseng and ginkgo biloba (known for immune enhancement and improving blood flow, respectively, in Chinese medicine) are favorite herbal additives in energy drinks. It's doubtful these products contain enough of these herbs to be effective. Since ginseng needs special handling to retain its medicinal properties, the chances of its survival after being dissolved in a sugary liquid are less than those of winning the lottery. On a positive note, it's fortunate for the unsuspecting consumer that the herbal concentration is weak, because medicinal herbs are just that, medicinal. Ginseng can interact with heart medications, antidepressants, and diuretics, and ginkgo biloba has blood-thinning and insulin-altering properties.

I tell teens who ask me about these drinks that if they are worried about congestive heart failure, irregular heartbeats, Alzheimer's, and erectile dysfunction (all common uses for these types of vitamins, minerals, and herbs), they should first see a doctor, then realize that these products are a matter of personal taste, not neccesarily health. To this, the college crowd tells me energy drinks make good cocktail mixers . . . need I say more?

SPORTS DRINKS

A better choice for energy and hydration is sports drinks—but only if you need them; otherwise they are nothing more than extra calories. For active people, sports drinks can prevent dehydration and help recharge muscles with much-needed carbohydrates.

Sports drinks are designed specifically for people who work out intensely for at least an hour a day. If you work out infrequently or not at all, stick to water. Each company has its own formulations, so read the ingredients carefully. For instance, some are made with a blend of various sugars designed for optimal absorption of fluids and carbohydrates, while others are simply HFCS. Also, look out for sugar alcohols, which can have a laxative effect—an unwanted workout companion.

JUICE LABELING

I will never forget the day in 1996 that I heard about the death of a sixteen-month-old Colorado girl and more than sixty other individuals' being stricken ill from Odwalla's unpasteurized apple juice. The company's products were a staple at our morning editorial meetings, and the staff at the Half Moon Bay company were well known for their spirited enterprise and good nature.

It's hard to quantify the grief we felt for the victims' families and company employees when we heard the news. To add to the internal strife, the law firm Marler Clark represented the victims' families (a company I held in high regard for their legal representation of victims of food-borne illness). The situation was like getting caught in the middle of the divorce of two respected people.

Secretly, many believed the personal and professional loss was too great to overcome and the company would close its doors forever. Sales plummeted 90% and the media reported that federal investigators were looking into whether the company had ignored earlier warnings about product safety. Company officials admitted in court a plea of ignorance, saying they had not adequately anticipated the risk for unpasteurized juices.

As plea deals, fines, and compensation to the victims' families were finalized in court, the company faced as best it could its responsibility to food safety. Products were recalled while Odwalla sought out experts and developed critical control measures including sanitation and flash pasteurization, a quick, high-temperature pasteurization process.

No amount of self-regulation could bring back the young girl who died or ease the suffering of the ill, but Odwalla's actions did set a higher standard for the fresh juice industry, which prevented such a tragedy from happening again in the packaged-juice market. As a result, federally mandated safety measures for agricultural and manufacturing practices were proposed along with a warning label for unpasteurized juices.

Even with the seriousness of the issue, reviews were mixed. During the comment period, the editorial staff where I worked heard from fresh juice manufacturers and associations that the warning label was alarmist and unnecessary and that pasteurization was too expensive for small presses to afford and the heat killed healthy enzymes in fresh juices.

The FDA stuck by the warning claim. The only concessions made were for juice bars and restaurants that press juice on-site and serve it by the glass (the FDA warns that on-site freshly pressed juices still pose health risks). Otherwise, all packaged juice must be pasteurized or carry the label:

> WARNING: *This product has not been pasteurized and, therefore, may contain harmful bacteria that can cause serious illness in children, the elderly, and persons with weakened immune systems.*

Portion Control   The next crisis to hit the juice market was the low-carb craze. Consumer fears about sugar sent sales plummeting—it was an unfortunate message. Juices are high in naturally occurring sugars but provide added benefits—if the portions are controlled. Fruits contain glucose, fructose, fiber, antioxidants, and a long list of vitamins, including A and C, potassium, and folic acid. The latest finds for healthy living include pomegranate and blueberry juice, which contain more antioxidants and polyphenols than even wine or grape juice.

It's the fiber in fruit that regulates the body's speed of sugar absorption. Take out the fiber and it's a quick shot of liquid energy, which is why sticking with a single serving is important. Calorie-for-calorie, one medium-sized apple has the same 120 calories as three-quarters cup of juice. Three medium-sized oranges have about 195 calories, which is how many it takes to squeeze out one cup of juice (110 calories).

Rather than fill a todder's sippee cup with an endless supply of juice or let your teenage son chug from the carton, measure it out to know what a single serving looks like. A serving for a child from one to four years is four to six ounces (half to three-quarters cup). For older children and adults, a single serving is six to eight ounces (three-quarters to one cup), which will fill a small juice glass to the rim.

For children and adults with sensitive stomachs, stick to low-sorbitol juices such as white grape and strawberry, raspberry, blueberry, and blackberry. Also, be cautious of juice drinks labeled as low in sugar, as they contain sugar alcohols, which can also cause stomach problems.

Last, be wary of products that say "made with fruit juices"; they're nothing more than sugar water with some vitamin C thrown in. Marketers might even add the word "natural," but don't give in; any product that uses the word "drink," "beverage," or "cocktail" is not 100% juice.

Functional Juices   If anything, the low-carb craze lit a fire under the juice industry to improve on a good thing with fortified juices that contain selenium, plant sterols, calcium, and vitamins E, C, and D. These nutrients are scientifically backed, making them popular among health-minded seniors and baby boomers, for antiaging, cancer-fighting, and bone-strengthening properties.

Buying fortified juices is a lot like choosing vitamins; look carefully at the ingredients. For instance, calcium citrate malate is better absorbed than other calcium sources. For the best heart health benefits look for juices with plant sterols that contain at least .8g per serving and have the following label: *"Foods containing at least 0.4 gram per serving of plant sterols, consumed twice a day with meals for a total daily intake of at least 0.8 gram, as part of a diet low in saturated fat and cholesterol, may reduce the risk of heart disease."* Finally, always shake the container, since many of the vitamins and mineral additives fall to the bottom of the carton.

Organic Juice   According to pesticide residue surveys, juices score more favorably than fresh fruit, as long as the consumer is an adult. Add in one small variable—a pint-sized child—and the equation expands from basic math to calculus. Pound for pound, young children eat more than adults, and as any parent will tell you, they eat the same foods over and over again. Juice is a favorite.

The last Consumers Union tests for pesticide residues (2000) gave children's three favorite fruit juices a relatively clean report card. Orange and grape juice residues pose a small risk, for domestic or imported brands. Apple juice has a higher risk depending on the country of origin—German and Chilean apple juice has the lowest risk, domestic juice was in the middle, while Chinese and Argentinian apple juice had the highest residue levels. Consumers Union found that apple juice pesticide residue is ten times higher than orange and grape juice residue, but the overall toxicity index is still low for pesticide residues. If your parenting style is cautious, consider adding organic juices to your child's drink choices. If nothing else, organic orange juice can contain 30% more vitamin C than conventional juice; that's without any fortification.

BOTTLED WATER

In the small Italian village I moved to Colorado from, the tap water was in such short supply that we didn't have running water in the middle of the day during the summer months. Water was plentiful in the winter, but the town's officials often posted *E. coli* warnings regarding the stressed and ancient aquaduct system. Year-round, I relied on bottled water for drinking. In the summer, cement cisterns slowly collected water in the middle of the night for bathing and clothes washing.

After years of showering and doing laundry at midnight and lugging cases of bottled water, it was a luxury in Colorado to drink tap water that was clean and tasted amazing. Even though our water comes from glaciers and mountain streams, Coloradans still love bottled water, as do many other Americans, who spend more than $9 billion per year on bottled water.

Americans drink bottled water for the convenience and the taste and because of concerns about water quality. Are the fears well founded? The decision to drink bottled water is skewed by nothing more than our perception that bottled is better. Neither bottle nor tap are perfect sources. Two separate agencies monitor water safety standards for tap and bottled water—the EPA oversees the water from the faucet, and bottled water falls under the category of food, which the FDA owns. The FDA categorizes water in these five categories:

Artesian water is from a well that is contained within an impervious layer of rock or sand, called an aquifer. The water level sits at a height above the aquifer.

Distilled/purified water is purified using distillation, a process that boils water and collects the steam. Deionizaton is a similar process. This type of water is commonly used in irons and humidifiers.

Mineral water contains no fewer than 250 ppm of dissolved trace elements and minerals, such as calcium, magnesium, and potassium.

Minerals cannot be added to this water; they must be naturally oc-
curing.

Sparkling water is effervescent at its source from naturally occurring carbon dioxide. During extraction, the carbon dioxide is separated from the water, which gets filtered, after which the carbon
dioxide is added back in. Seltzer and club soda are considered soft
drinks, not sparkling water.

Well water comes from a hole in the ground that taps into a water
aquifer.

Is the bottled-water industry doing any better than the EPA for
quality standards? Pardon the pun, but it's a wash, primarily because
at least 25% of bottled water is tap water. If you think bottled water
tastes better than water from the faucet, that is because most companies use ozone gas rather than chlorine as a disinfectant. If you think
bottled water is safer, consider that it took until 2005 for the FDA to
finally get around to setting standards for mandatory arsenic testing
for bottled water. Conversely, the lead levels for bottled water are
lower than the EPA's for tap water, 5 ppb as compared to 15 ppb, respectively. Again, it's a wash.

The most common phrases on bottled water say the water was filtered using a "highly sophisticated purification process." This highly
sophisticated process may be no different from the same process used
for your tap water. That makes for a really expensive tap water—as
high as twelve dollars a gallon.

Ultra-purification water is the latest filtration process to hit the
bottled-water market. Companies that sell the water claim to remove all
arsenic, bacteria, chlorine, chromium 6, fluoride, lead, and pesticides.

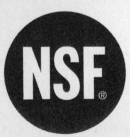

There is currently only one voluntary labeling program that is an extra guarantee that the
water bottler meets, or exceeds, FDA standards
for safety. An independent, not-for-profit organization called NSF International, as noted by
a tiny NSF circular seal, certifies water brands
(see the company Web site, www.nsf.org, for
specific brands). The program inspects each

facility annually, unannounced, to make certain the company meets appropriate federal regulations.

Overall, studies that compared bacterial levels in tap and bottled water show that neither source is perfectly free of contaminants. The key difference is transparency, since municipal water utilities are required to tell you if there is a problem via your monthly bill. If you want to know more about your local water quality, go to the EPA Web site and look up the report for your community; if it's not there, make a phone call to the utility company.

FDA says the current recall system is more than sufficient to protect consumers from problems with bottled water. A recent recall illustrates that the system has some flaws. In summer of 2006 a widespread recall for bottled water was announced that affected numerous private label brands from supermarkets in New York. The water was supplied by Springbrook Springs in Concord, New York, and contained an unacceptable level of bromate (as high as 28 ppb). FDA limits are 10 ppb; over a very long time frame (seventy years) it may be cancer-causing. FDA said in this instance there was no immediate risk to consumer health.

The International Bottled Water Association, the industry's voice regarding such issues, released a statement saying the recall "demonstrated the protective nature of FDA bottled-water regulation." This argument might hold true if the actual bottler or even FDA had discovered the mistake and called for the recall. However, in this case, the high bromate levels were discovered by two men who pulled the products from store shelves. A water product-development consultant, Larry Alibrandi, and his lawyer, Ross Getman, tested water bottles within a one-week sell-by date in July 2006 and discovered the problem. As of this writing, they are continuing to pull water from central New York stores and test for bromate (Alibrandi and Getman were also the whistleblowers for the soft-drink benzene case).

So how does the bromate get in the water? That is the other disconcerting fact. The water bottler puts it there. Here is the chain of events: During the "purification" process, calcium chloride, which contains bromide, is added to flavor the mineral, spring, or tap water, which may have already been purified by municipalities (why water needs flavor, I'm not sure). Then, ozone gas is pumped through the water. This process oxidizes the water and creates bromate. If done improperly, the bromate levels may exceed FDA's 10-ppb legal limit.

The last factor to consider when buying bottled water is the amount of plastic used to make water bottles. Most water bottles are made from polyethylene terephthalate (PET), which is derived from crude oil. Meeting the increased demand for just the bottles for all that water requires more than 1.5 million barrels of oil yearly—the same amount of fuel for nearly 100,000 cars for the same time frame. In addition, most water bottles end up in landfills, which only adds to the problem. Again, a water filter may be a better solution than bottled water.

Vitamin Water   Water spiked with vitamins? Mmmm. These drinks were designed for boomers who were being dragged tooth and nail into old age by Old Man Time. On the pro side, I suppose they are better than an HFCS-sweetened drink. On the con, is this really the fountain of youth or a gimmick?

When Consumer Labs, an independent dietary supplement testing company, ran four vitamin waters through their laboratories, they discovered that only one had the labeled amount of vitamin C. That's not surprising, since vitamin C breaks down very easily when exposed to air. I'll leave it up to you to decide if the price for sweetened vitamin water is worth it when a better outcome can be derived from a plain glass of water and a multivitamin pill.

Bottom Line

I have decided that "personal responsibility" is the new buzzword for "it's not my problem." While I was finishing this chapter, it was announced that the global obesity rate has reached pandemic proportions. Who is responsible? No one and everyone, depending on whom you ask.

I was recently interviewed for a publication (of which I am a member), by Les Dames d'Escoffier, a nonprofit group that works to provide scholarships to women interested in culinary fields and grants to support school garden projects and healthy school-lunch programs.

I was asked, "How will [my] women readers influence those food and culinary trends?" Here is part of my answer.

For most women, food is personal. Women recognize that food fuels the body, gives children life, maintains health, and provides a great deal of pleasure—whether cooking at home or dining out. Forget pork-barrel spenders, politicians, well-connected lobbyists, and powerful corporations. Women have always brandished the power to generate the most change in our food system because more often than not women hold the purse strings. Women can transform our food policies, farming practices, and the health of the nation by voting with their dollar at grocery stores, farmers' markets, restaurants, and even their children's schools. My dream is that at least one day every month, all American mothers will simultaneously not give their child lunch money and instead pack a healthy lunch as an example of just how much influence the American mother quietly holds over this country's school-lunch system. Imagine.

I am hopeful that food companies will recognize how their decisions influence the country's and the world's health. I am also hopeful that the types of products sold within school bounds are being monitored, and that school districts will see that this is not enough. Mandatory physical education for all grades, whether it's skateboarding, bike riding, or just taking a walk during school hours, is necessary for long-term good health. I am hopeful that parents will also take a more active role to provide healthy meals to young children and get back in the kitchen with their older kids. Personal responsibility is a shared responsibility.

Shop Healthy and Live Well

When I see friends in the grocery store, the first thing they often say is, "Don't look in my shopping cart," as if I am a grocery store hall monitor. Believe me, there are days I feel the urge to load up on Oreos, Cheetos, and Apple Cinnamon Cheerios, just a few of my forbidden favorites. On *most* occasions, I refrain. However, I hope from this book you've realized that I am not a food enforcement officer, rather a mom, wife, and journalist, looking for the best way to navigate our complicated food system.

I can tell you that if you read up on the history of the USDA and FDA, you'll realize the farming and food industry has been struggling with the very same issues since their inceptions. To illustrate, here is something Abraham Lincoln said during his campaign for president: "Populations must increase rapidly and ere long the most valuable of all the arts will be the art of deriving a comfortable subsistence from the smallest area of soil." Depending on one's perspective today, Lincoln's words could reflect an interest in concentrated farming methods or an environmentally biodiverse agricultural system.

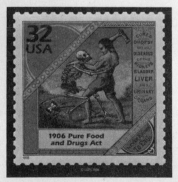

In the early 1900s, Dr. Harvey W. Wiley, a former Civil War soldier and Purdue chemistry professor and appointee as the first head of the Bureau of Chemistry (the predecessor agency to the FDA), faced the same push and pull of food marketing versus consumer safety and transparency. Wiley's very public clashes easily mirror the FDA's modern era debates, including loose labeling, false advertising, and the safety of preservatives, food coloring, and artificial sweeteners. At the time, the laws lacked enough teeth for Wiley to make substantial changes. The Food and Drugs Act of 1906 was the only law to regulate food and drugs. It gave no authority to the government to test ingredients for safety and prove what was actually in the product. Advertisers could make any claims, regardless of truth, and no scientist could prove otherwise.

Wiley fought for the consumer, especially on two chemicals—sodium benzoate, a preservative in canned foods, and saccharin, the alternative sweetener being passed off as sugar on food labels. It's been more than one hundred years; do these two particular ingredients sound familiar (see the beverage chapter)? Upon Wiley's retirement in 1912, many businesspeople who fought him so forcefully admitted that he had been correct in many of his actions and opinions.

In retrospect, each administration since then has adopted or vetoed numerous policy changes that can be celebrated or brooded over, depending on one's political and food preferences. If nothing else, these spirited debates motivate entrepreneurs to improve the quality and safety and expand the choices of our food. The following history lesson is a synopsis of the most significant changes in food policy in the last seventy-five years.

Food, Drug, and Cosmetic Act In 1933 Walter G. Campbell, a new hire under Wiley's administration and then head of the FDA, along with the USDA and the Consumers' Research Group (now Consumers Union), introduced the bill to take decision making out of the courts and into the laboratory. Today the trend of using the courts to solve food arguments and force self-regulation is again popular.

Naturally, food and drug companies wanted no part of the FDC Act. Letter-writing campaigns accused the FDA of being more interested in the public than food and drug businesses. The FDA and USDA fought back with their own display of products that exemplified the corporate recklessness. Opium and morphine could be ordered by mail; crystals and salts advertised to cure high blood pressure,

rheumatism, and constipation killed hundreds of unsuspecting customers. Toxic weight-loss products marketed to women caused an epidemic of cataracts, blindness, kidney, liver and blood disorders, and
death. Less serious issues of food fraud included selling corn syrup as
maple syrup and strawberry jams with no strawberries. During the
congressional hearings, a reporter named the exhibit the "Chamber of
Horrors." He may have been one of the few journalists in attendance,
since news coverage of the act was scarcely a whisper.

Delaney Clause   This 1959 amendment to the Food, Drug and Cosmetic Act required manufacturers to prove the safety of pesticide
residues, food additives, and color additives in processed foods (not raw
foods). For the first time, no substance could be legally introduced into
the U.S. food supply unless there was conclusive proof that it was safe.
The Delaney Clause opened up the ongoing debate about how to determine a safe level for possible carcinogens in food additives, colors, and
pesticides. The same year the Delaney Clause passed, the USDA culled
the seven basic food groups down to four—fruits and vegetables, milk,
meat, and breads/cereals. Nearly fifty years later the food pyramid is
still being revised to try to convince us to eat better.

The Food Quality and Protection Act   In 1996, this act amended
the Delaney Clause to modernize food safety law, which unified safety
standards for processed and raw foods with the intention of setting
safer pesticide tolerances to protect pregnant women, infants, and
children.

Nutrition Labeling and Education Act of 1990 (NLEA)   You may
not remember it, but earlier in your lifetime the Nutrition Facts Panel
on the side of the box, bag, or package wasn't there. It's largely taken
for granted now, but getting it there took some work. Prior to legislation called the Nutrition Labeling and Education Act of 1990 that required the panel, the food industry had health claims on as many as
40% of its products and not all the information was there to inform
but instead to persuade.

At the time, FDA commissioner David Kessler—an issues-oriented, public policy–minded person—was the perfect man to sort out the food labeling quagmire. Kessler is often compared to Wiley because he took the FDA's responsibility of regulation to heart, a brave move during a political atmosphere of deregulation in the Reagan administration. Kessler's first public speech to the Food and Drug Law Institute made that very clear: "The FDA is the regulator, and you should know that I have no problem stating that fact. The FDA must stand for, it must embody, strong and judicious enforcement . . ."

It's not surprising that strict regulators like Wiley and Kessler didn't always get along with powerful food lobbyists and their congressional representatives, though in this century I see the most promise, because instead of change being driven by courts and legislation, consumers are gaining control of the steering wheel. Regardless of whether the FDA, the USDA, or powerful food associations agree or disagree with the methods used to grow or raise GM foods, farmed salmon, or livestock with truly natural or organic food production methods, consumers are voting with their dollars. As long as entrepreneurs and corporate food giants see monetary value in better-managed farming policies and manufacturing practices, the number of food choices that use fewer pesticides and drugs and more stringent animal welfare guidelines will continue to increase. My hope is that in time all consumers, not just the well-to-do, can afford foods grown with these methods.

There are more than enough books, newspaper and magazine articles, white papers, and reports out there about the condition of American farms, ranches, and meat processors. And an ever-growing number say how we need to get closer to our food sources, reduce food miles, and boycott companies and retailers that don't meet utopian standards for organic agriculture.

As I said in the beginning of this book, while these ideologies are sometimes well-meaning, they can be taken to the extreme. On paper these concepts and investigative writings are very informative, but undoubtedly within at least three hours of reading you will be hungry and/or your child will be hungry and you will have to find something to eat. What will you do? Go out back and milk your cow or harvest some of your organic produce or head to the grocery store?

If you are like me, it's the latter. Other than the fact that your Home Owners' Association and neighbors would take issue with the cow idea, most of us cannot rearrange our entire lives or change the weather to buy *only* from small local farms all year round. I believe the new term for people who adopt this routine is "locavores." While I wholeheartedly support Colorado agriculture, my kids would put a sign in the yard that says "Kids for Rent, Inquire Within" if by January we were eating only Colorado-grown pinto beans and Boulder County goat cheese. Luckily, the organic rules don't specify how far a food must travel to be certified.

This idea is not new—for the past twenty years the pioneers of the organic food industry have wrestled with issues like how organic is organic. Over late-night Scotch parties at trade shows these agricultural visionaries pondered whether there should be such a food as organic Twinkies or what would happen if they got what they wished for— widespread acceptance of organic foods by consumers of all types, not just the chosen few who were religious followers. We are here; that day has arrived.

Much of what I see going on in the food world is very similar to the dietary supplement boom of the 1990s, when people were very hopeful that they could throw away their doctor's phone number and turn solely to herbs and dietary supplements for preventative health and to treat illness. While there are pockets of people who still thrive by using only alternative health-care providers, most find they need an integrative approach, one that combines an assortment of experts—M.D.s, acupuncturists, massage therapists, and chiropractors.

Today we are as likely to take an over-the-counter pain reliever and make an appointment with our chiropractor as we are to buy an organic apple from New Zealand, a hunk of strong aged cheese from a local dairy, and a diet soft drink. As always, once the revolutionaries on both sides of the barn have their say, most consumers will find their comfort zone squarely in the middle.

Besides, the American shopper doesn't need any more angst and guilt added to his or her day. Our children are better served by parents, relatives, and friends who live life in balance, rather than feeling pressured and overworked to meet the expectations of others who choose to live a different lifestyle. I hope that my book has conveyed this message. Above all, my wish is for you is to shop healthy and live well.

ADDENDUM

Since completing the book, some notable events have taken place that deserve a brief comment.

CHAPTER 1. GREENER ACRES WITHOUT CHANGING YOUR ADDRESS OR YOUR POLITICS

In mid-October 2006, there were more than 199 people sickened (102 hospitalizations, 3 deaths) from bagged spinach tainted with *E. coli* (0157:H7). The source was traced back to four fields in Monterey and San Benito counties in California. The suspected causes are livestock farms polluting water sources and the region's susceptibility to frequent flooding. Since the mid-1990s, there have been nineteen different foodborne-illness outbreaks from this region—for the very same reason. Uncontaminated spinach came in contact with *E. coli* at the primary processing plant, owned by Natural Selection Foods, which processes greens from farms outside their control. To counter the problem, Natural Selection will now test all produce that enters the processing facility (FDA is calling for tighter food safety measures in the fields). These measures will hopefully reduce exposure, but understand that this type of bacteria cannot be washed away. Cooking is the only fail-safe way to prevent illness from *E. coli* 0517:H7. For persons with chronic health problems, such as kidney disease, it is well advised to cook spinach if the source is unknown; otherwise, buy from farms that have a well-documented safety program in place (to date, no state other than California has reported widespread problems).

CHAPTER 2. SLAUGHTERHOUSE SEMANTICS: BEEF, PORK, AND LAMB

The FDA announced in October 2006 that all food processors and manufacturers of products (foods, supplements, cosmetics) made from, with, or containing materials from cattle must keep extensive records to prove that their products are not made using prohibited animal parts that could further the spread of BSE.

CHAPTER 5. SEA OF LABELS: FISH

The Pregnancy Outcomes and Community Health study (POUCH) analyzed the diets of 1,204 pregnant women who ate fish—those who ate more had higher blood levels of mercury than non–fish eaters (average was .29 ppm). Authors noted that 44 of these women had premature births, but added that more research is needed to prove if there is a connection to diet. Comments about the study advised pregnant women to stay within the FDA guidelines. In addition, the National Research Council recommended that Americans eat fish at lease twice a week for optimum heart health, but vary the types to minimize mercury exposure.

President Bush directed the State and Commerce departments to support sustainable fishing practices worldwide, and specifically oppose bottom trawling. The directive came the day before a UN vote to ban the practice. Pundits called it a political move to gain support from key state senators and U.S. allies that support the ban. Say what you will, but hopefully something positive will come from better U.S. support for ocean conservation. In the same time period, researchers discovered that a blend of vegetable and fish oil used for farmed salmon feed can replace 75% of fish oil without adversely affecting taste and omega-3 fatty acid composition. The new science could help reduce reliance on small fish stocks for salmon feed.

CHAPTER 6. DAIRY DAZE

Since completing the dairy chapter, I visited Aurora's new dairy in Eastern Colorado, which is owned (and leased back to Aurora) by a Colorado dairy farming family. It is a $10 million model of sustainability with more than ample pasture space. Neighboring farmers are so impressed they are converting their dairies and land to organic production. Horizon is also in the process of redesigning the Idaho farm, but I have not yet seen the farm to report on the changes.

CHAPTER 7. GRAINS OF TRUTH: PASTA, BREAD, CEREAL, AND GRAINS

The following is a response to my inquiry to the American Heart Association Certification program staff about why cereals with high sugar and low trans-fats levels are allowed to carry the AHA seal:

> **Sugars:** *There simply isn't scientific data that proves sugar plays a role in heart disease. The federal government regulations for coronary heart disease health claims identify two criteria to determine whether a coronary heart disease health claim may be made for a food product: dietary saturated fat and cholesterol. To be eligible for the Food Certification Program, a food product must meet the American Heart Association's criteria for being "low" in saturated fat and cholesterol. There also is a disqualifier for sodium, if the sodium content is too high (more than 480mg for individual foods). Sugar is not a criterion or disqualifier because there is not sufficient scientific evidence to show that sugar is a risk factor for coronary heart disease. The FDA and American Heart Association are in agreement on the sugar issue. Although sugar has not been directly linked to heart disease, the American Heart Association recommends a diet moderate in added sugar as part of an overall eating plan for healthy individuals over the age of two. People who are trying to achieve a healthy weight or who want to prevent weight gain should limit their intake of foods containing a lot of excess sugar.*
>
> **Trans fat:** *At this time the Food Certification Program does not include criteria for trans fatty acid levels. To date, the FDA has not established a Daily Value for it. The FDA extended the comment period for the ANPRM (advanced notice of proposed rulemaking) for trans fatty acid labeling (which ended on June 18, 2004). We continue to track the emerging science on this topic,*

and should federal regulations for coronary heart health claims change to include trans fatty acid levels, the Food Certification Program will include them in its criteria.

CHAPTER 8. CHANGE YOUR OIL

In October 2006, FDA approved a qualified health claim for its ability to reduce the risk of heart disease because of its unsaturated fat content. In a nutshell, the claim recommends substituting 1½ tablespoons of canola oil daily for saturated fat and not to increase the number of calories eaten in a day.

CHAPTER 13. AISLE OF DENIAL: CARBONATED AND SWEETENED BEVERAGES

A major gap in school nutrition is that USDA has no legal oversight for foods sold outside the school lunch program. Five of the major snack food companies—Kraft Foods, Mars, PepsiCo, Dannon, and Campbell Soup Company—are working with former president Bill Clinton and the AHA to reformulate snacks sold in schools. In addition, the Child Nutrition and WIC Reauthorization Act now requires that schools participating in its lunch or breakfast programs agree to a wellness policy that sets nutritional standards for all foods sold in schools.

The purpose of *Eating Between the Lines* is to help you become a discerning shopper. This top-ten list and the wallet-sized shopping cards are reminders of the types of labels you may come across in the grocery store and what they mean.

Top Ten Labeling Reminders

1. **Beef:** The USDA definition of "natural" is about food processing, not the way the animal was raised. For restrained use of hormones and antibiotics look for organic, beyond natural, and certified animal welfare brands.

2. **Poultry and Eggs:** Don't buy into the "no-hormone" trap and pay more for products that make such claims. Look for brands that at the very least use no human-grade antibiotics.

3. **Seafood:** No matter what, eat at least two servings of fish per week. For mercury- and PCB-safe brands look for safety testing symbols.

4. **Dairy:** If you prefer to avoid rGBH-treated milk, look for the "No Growth Hormones Used" labels or buy organic.

5. **Extra-Virgin Olive Oil:** PAGED: *price* ($12–20/liter), *acidity* (less than .8g), *geography* (single country or region), *extra-virgin* for the most health properties and flavor, *date*.

6. **Health Claims:** No amount of marketing can make an unhealthy product healthy.

7. **Coffee:** Fair Trade Certified and specialty coffee sellers with social welfare programs are a necessary cause in today's coffee marketplace.

8. **Cereals and Snacks:** Use a critical eye to find products that are high in fiber and low in sugar, and have absolutely no trans fats.

9. **Beverages:** One twelve-ounce sweetened drink has at least nine teaspoons of HFCS or sugar.

10. **Moderation:** Nutrient content claims are for a 2,000-calorie diet. If this is more than you need to consume, pay attention to the portion size, calories, and percentage of saturated fats.

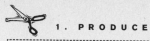

1. PRODUCE

Fruit and Vegetable Pesticide Residues				
Most Residues		**Kids' Favorites That Use Organo-phosphates (OPs)**	**Least Residues**	
FRUITS	**VEGETABLES**		**FRUITS**	**VEGETABLES**
Apples	Celery	Apples	Kiwi	Asparagus
Cherries	Potatoes	Melon, imported	Mango	Avocado
Grapes,	Spinach	Carrots	Bananas	Onions
imported	Bell Peppers	Green Beans	Papaya	Broccoli
Nectarines	Lettuce	Potatoes	Pineapple	Cauliflower
Pears	(winter)	Tomatoes		Peas (sweet)
Peaches		Winter Squash		Corn (sweet)
Raspberries				
Strawberries				

Sources: Environmental Working Group; USDA Pesticide Data Program 2003; Environmental Protection Agency

Least Pesticide Residues of All:

2. MEAT, POULTRY

	Beef and Bison	Pork	Lamb	Chicken
No Added Hormones	USDA ORGANIC · CERTIFIED HUMANE RAISED & HANDLED · American Humane Association FREE FARMED CERTIFIED · DEMETER CERTIFIED BIODYNAMIC® **Beyond Natural** · American Grassfed **All Bison**	N/A	N/A	N/A
No Antibiotics	USDA ORGANIC · DEMETER CERTIFIED BIODYNAMIC® · American Grassfed **Beyond Natural** **All Bison**	same	same	same
No Human-Grade Antibiotics or Limited Antibiotics	American Humane Association FREE FARMED CERTIFIED · CERTIFIED HUMANE RAISED & HANDLED · American Grassfed	Pork Quality Assurance (PQA Plus)	same as beef	Foster Farms, Gold Kist, Perdue, and Tyson; for other brands call the company

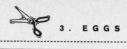

3. EGGS

Eco-Friendly	No Antibiotics	Egg Safety
USDA ORGANIC; CERTIFIED HUMANE RAISED & HANDLED; American Humane Association; DEMETER CERTIFIED BIODYNAMIC®; FREE FARMED CERTIFIED; American Grassfed **Beyond Natural**	same	Egg Quality Assurance Programs; Pasteurized; Irradiated; mind the dates and handling instructions

4. SEAFOOD

Low-Mercury Labels	Stewardship	Safety
Safe Harbor CERTIFIED SEAFOOD www.safeharborfoods.com SEAFOOD SAFE 10 4oz. Servings Adult/Month (or 5 - 8oz.) *www.seafoodsafe.com Lab Tested for Mercury & PCBs*	MARINE STEWARDSHIP COUNCIL© U.S. Department of Commerce Dolphin Safe **Monterey Bay** **Seafood Watch**	Pay attention to appearance and dates; safe handling

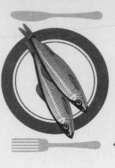

MERCURY IN FISH

A Guide for Women and Children

NRDC NATURAL RESOURCES DEFENSE COUNCIL
THE EARTH'S BEST DEFENSE
www.nrdc.org

EATING CANNED TUNA SAFELY

WHITE ALBACORE		CHUNK LIGHT	
If you weigh:	Don't eat more than	If you weigh:	Don't eat more than
11 lbs	1 can/4 months	11 lbs	1 can/6 weeks
22 lbs	1 can/2 months	22 lbs	1 can/23 days
33 lbs	1 can/5 weeks	33 lbs	1 can/2 weeks
44 lbs	1 can/4 weeks	44 lbs	1 can/12 days
55 lbs	1 can/3 weeks	55 lbs	1 can/9 days
66 lbs	1 can/3 weeks	66 lbs	1 can/8 days
77 lbs	1 can/3 weeks	77 lbs	1 can/week
88 lbs	1 can/2 weeks	88 lbs	1 can/6 days
99 lbs	1 can/2 weeks	99 lbs	1 can/5 days
110 lbs	1 can/12 days	110 lbs	1 can/5 days
121 lbs	1 can/11 days	121 lbs	1 can/4 days
132 lbs	1 can/10 days	132 lbs	1 can/4 days
143 lbs	1 can/9 days	143 lbs	1 can/4 days
154 lbs	1 can/9 days	154 lbs	1 can/3 days
165+ lbs	1 can/8 days	165+ lbs	1 can/3 days

This guide is just one of the tools in NRDC's mercury protection toolkit.

See the NRDC Web site for:

- Tips about mercury in sushi and sportfish, and details about all of NRDC's mercury guides

- A calculator you can use to estimate how much mercury you may be eating

- Maps of mercury sources and state-by-state mercury warnings for anglers

- Information on how mercury pollution gets into the environment and into fish

- An online action center where you can help stop mercury pollution

www.nrdc.org/mercury

Oct 2004

Eating fish is good for you, right?

It can be. But some fish is high in mercury, a chemical that can cause serious health problems, especially for children and pregnant women.

If you are pregnant or planning to become pregnant, use this guide to see what amounts of fish caught and sold commercially are safe to eat.

To gauge safe amounts for your children, reduce the portion sizes.

Information in this guide is based on the FDA's test results for mercury in fish and the EPA's determination of safe levels of mercury for children and women of reproductive age (no guidelines exist for other adults).

HIGHEST MERCURY

AVOID EATING:

Grouper*	Shark*
Marlin*	Swordfish*
Mackerel (king)	Tilefish*
Orange roughy*	

HIGH MERCURY

EAT NO MORE THAN THREE 6-OZ. SERVINGS PER MONTH:

Bass (saltwater)*
Bluefish
Croaker
Halibut*
Lobster (American/Maine)
Sea trout
Tuna (canned, white albacore)
Tuna (fresh bluefin, ahi)

LOWER MERCURY

EAT NO MORE THAN SIX 6-OZ. SERVINGS PER MONTH:

Carp
Cod*
Crab (blue)
Crab (Dungeness)
Crab (snow)
Mahi Mahi
Monkfish*
Perch (freshwater)
Skate
Snapper*
Tuna (canned, chunk light)
Tuna (fresh Pacific albacore)

LOWEST MERCURY

ENJOY THESE FISH:

Anchovies	Oysters
Butterfish	Perch (saltwater)
Calamari (squid)	Pollock
Catfish	Salmon#
Caviar (farmed)	Sardines
Clams	Scallops
Crab (king)*	Shad
Crawfish/crayfish	Shrimp*
Flounder*	Sole
Haddock*	Sturgeon (farmed)
Hake	Tilapia
Herring	Trout (freshwater)
Lobster (spiny/rock)	Whitefish

Farmed salmon may contain PCBs, manufactured chemicals with serious long-term health effects. (PCBs were banned in the U.S. in the 1970s but remain in the environment.)

* Fish in trouble! These fish are perilously low in numbers or are caught using environmentally destructive methods.

Author's note: See chapter 5 for clarification on "fish in trouble."

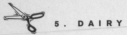

5. DAIRY

No Growth Hormones	Fat Grams per Cup	Quality
"No Growth Hormones Used" USDA ORGANIC CERTIFIED HUMANE RAISED & HANDLED American Humane Association FREE FARMED CERTIFIED DEMETER CERTIFIED BIODYNAMIC® American Grassfed	Whole Milk—8g 2%–4.7g 1%–2.6g Skim—.5g or less	*Live & Active Cultures REAL

6. PROCESSED FOODS, CEREALS, GRAINS

Whole Grain, Low Glycemic Index	Healthy Cereals	Whole Grains	Eat Healthy Snacks	Avoid
100% WHOLE GRAIN 16g or more per serving WholeGrainsCouncil.org EAT 48g OR MORE OF WHOLE GRAINS DAILY LOW GLYCEMIC WASHINGTON, D.C. CERTIFIED BY THE GLYCEMIC RESEARCH INSTITUTE ®	5g fiber or more 5g sugar or less 3g protein or more	Barley Buckwheat Bulgur Corn *Farro* Kamut Millet Oats Quinoa Rice Rye Wild Rice	Liquid Vegetable Oils No Trans Fats Reduced Saturated Fat Low Sugar 100% Whole Grains Portion Control	High-Sodium Snacks Trans Fats Saturated Fats Empty-Calorie Snacks— High Sugar and Re-fined Flours

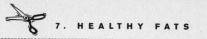

7. HEALTHY FATS

Healthy Oils	Gourmet/Quality Labels
Canola Nut Extra-Virgin Olive Enova Flaxseed Hemp High Oleic Safflower and Sunflower	*Appellation d'Origine Contrôllée (AOC), Denominación de Origen Protegida (DOP), Denominazione di Origine Protetta (DOP), Helleniz Foreign Trade Board (HEPO)*

8. COFFEE AND TEA

Eco-Friendly	Socially Conscious
USDA ORGANIC · BIRD FRIENDLY · RAINFOREST ALLIANCE CERTIFIED · NATIONAL WILDLIFE FEDERATION	FAIR TRADE CERTIFIED STARBUCKS CAFE COFFEE KIDS® GROUNDS FOR HOPE www.coffeekids.org

9. SUGARS AND SWEETENERS

Sweeteners	Sugar Substitutes	Portions
Sucrose	Acesulfame-K	4g sugar or HFCS=1 tsp.
Cane Sugar	Aspartame	12-ounce soda=40g or 9¾
Invert Sugar	Erythritol	tsps. sweeteners
High-Fructose	Neotame	Single serving of juice:
Corn Syrup	Polydextrose	4–6 oz.=½–¾ cup
(HFCS)	Saccharin	6–8 oz.=¾–1 cup
Dextrose	Tagatose	
Fructose	Talin	
Stevia	Sugar Alcohols—lactitol, sorbitol, mannitol, xylitol	

10. PORTION SIZES

Daily Recommendations:	1 Portion Equivalent
2 cups or 4–5 servings of each	**FRUITS AND VEGETABLES** ½ cup = 1 medium fruit fist size or the size of a baseball ½ cup raw or cooked fist-size serving of leafy greens
5.5 ounces	**MEATS, POULTRY, EGGS, BEANS, NUTS** 1 ounce meat = size of a hockey puck or deck of cards 1 egg ¼ cup cooked beans walnut-size ball of peanut butter or heaping tablespoon
3 1-cup and/or 1-ounce servings	**DAIRY** 1 cup milk, yogurt, or alternative milk product 1 ounce cheese = size of 2 dice
6 teaspoons	**OILS** 1 tsp.–1 tbs. low-fat mayo 2 tablespoons light salad dressing
267 calories or 3.5 teaspoons solid fat 8 teaspoons sugar	**SOLID FATS AND SUGARS** A little more than 1 tablespoon One 8-ounce sweetened drink (the half-can size)

SELECTED BIBLIOGRAPHY

"100% Grassfed Ruminant Program: Measuring, Standards & Requirements," American Grassfed Association, February 28, 2005.

"ABC Airs Pro Genetic Engineering Message," *The Natural Foods Merchandiser*, August 2001.

Abelson, Jenn. "Got Organic? Demand Lifts Vermont Dairies," *The Boston Globe*, June 19, 2006.

Adams, Noah, and Bob Moon. "Marketplace Report: Wal-Mart's Organic Food Push, Day to Day," National Public Radio, May 12, 2006.

Albert, Christine M., M.D., Hannia Campos, Ph.D., et al. "Blood Levels of Long Chain n-3 Fatty Acids and the Risk of Sudden Death," *The New England Journal of Medicine*, 346, no. 15 (2002).

"Aldermen Turn Up Heat over Meat Treatment: Meat Industry Says Carbon Monoxide Safe as a Preservative," NBC5 News (Chicago, Illinois), June 7, 2006.

Allison, Melissa. "PCC Says Horizon Milk Will Be Pulled," *The Seattle Times*, August 11, 2006.

Annual Fish Stock Reports, National Oceanic and Atmospheric Administration (NOAA), U.S. Department of Commerce.

"Atkins Nutritionals Files for Bankruptcy," Associated Press, August 1, 2005.

Barboza, David. "Monsanto Sues Dairy in Maine Over Label's Remarks on Hormones," *The New York Times*, July 12, 2003.

Benbrook, Charles. "GM Crops Increase Pesticide Use: Impacts of Genetically Engineered Crops on Pesticide Use in the United States: The First Eight Years," BioTech, InfoNet, Technical Paper, no. 6, November 2003, at www.i-sis.org.uk.

————, Edward Groth III, Ph.D., et al. "Pesticide Residues in Conventional, IPM-grown, and Organic Foods: Insights from the Three Data Sets," released by Consumers Union, *Food Additives and Contaminants*, 19, no. 5 (2001): 427–46.

Benedictus, Leo. "How Can You Tell if Your Meat Is Organic?" *The Guardian*, May 16, 2006.

Boyle, Matthew. "The Man Who Fixed Kellogg Stale Offerings. Soggy Profits. Carlos Gutierrez Inherited Both When He Got the Top Job at the Cereal Giant. But Look at It Now," *Fortune* magazine, September 6, 2004.

Brady, Jeff. "Farmers Say Mega-Dairies Milk the Organic System," *All Things Considered*, National Public Radio, Washington, D.C., May 7, 2006.

Bren, Linda. "Antibiotic Resistance from Down on the Chicken Farm," *FDA Consumer* magazine, January–February 2001.

Brody, Jane. "Facing Biotech Foods Without the Fear Factor," *The New York Times*, January 11, 2005.

Brubaker, Harold. "Lancaster County Egg Farm Is Cited for Animal Cruelty," *Philadelphia Inquirer*, January 10, 2006.

Budgar, Laurie. "Battle Churns Over Organic Milk," *The Natural Foods Merchandiser*, March 1, 2006.

———. "Can Farmed Seafood Be Sustainable?" *The Natural Foods Merchandiser*, August 1, 2005.

Burros, Marian. "Poultry Industry Quietly Cuts Back on Antibiotic Use," *The New York Times*, February 10, 2002.

———. "Which Cut Is Older? (It's a Trick Question)," *The New York Times*, February 21, 2006.

"Calcium and Osteoporosis, 21CFR101.72, Guidance for Industry: Significant Scientific Agreement in the Review of Health Claims for Conventional Foods and Dietary Supplements," U.S. Department of Health and Human Services, Center for Food Safety and Applied Nutrition, FDA, December 22, 1999.

"Can Organic and Biotech Coexist? Biotech and Organic Crops Can Coexist with Clear and Cohesive Rules," Pew Initiative on Food and Biotechnology, *Roundtable*, 2, no. 6 (2002).

Cavadini, Claude, Anna Maria Siega-Riz, et al. "U.S. Adolescent Food Intake Trends from 1965 to 1996," *Western Journal of Medicine*, 173, no. 6 (2000).

Chea, Terence. "Organic Farms See Growth on More Demand," Associated Press, *San Francisco Chronicle*, May 30, 2006.

"City Council Airs Beef About Red Meat, Alderman Attempts to Ban Meat Treated with Carbon Monoxide," NBC5 News, March 23, 2006.

"Consumer Rights Group Warns of False Claims," *China Daily*, March 15, 2005.

Cox, James. "What's in a Name," *USA Today*, September 9, 2003.

"Dairy Groups Upset at WTO Talks Failure," *FoodNavigator.com*, July 7, 2006.

Davis, Donald, Ph.D., Melvin D. Epp, Ph.D., and Hugh Riordan, M.D. "Changes in USDA Food Composition Data for 43 Garden Crops, 1950–1999," *Journal of the American College of Nutrition*, 23, no. 6 (2004).

"Deal Briefs, Buyouts," Venture Economics (www.ventureeconomics.com), July 4, 2005.

"A Decade In: Is GM Winning Hearts and Minds?" *FoodNavigator.com*, January 18, 2006.

Derby, Brenda M., and Alan S. Levy. "Working Paper No. 1: Effects of Strength of Science Disclaimers on the Communication Impacts of Health Claims," Division of Social Sciences, Office of Regulations and Policy, Center for Food Safety and Applied Nutrition, FDA, September 2005.

"Dietary Alpha-linolenic Acid Reduces Inflammatory and Lipid Cardiovascular Risk Factors in Hypercholesterolemic Men and Women," *Journal of Nutrition*, 134, no. 11 (2004).

Dohoo, I. R., L. DesCoteaux, et al. "A Meta-Analysis Review of the Effects of Recombinant Bovine Somatotropin," *Canadian Journal of Veterinary Research*, 67, no. 4, October 2003.

"E.U. Bans Battery Cages," BBC News, January 28, 1999.

"Europe Clears Pepsi Merger," *Financial Times*, February 3, 2001.

"Evaluation of the Potential for Bovine Spongiform Encephalopathy in the United States," November 30, 2001, revised October 31, 2002, second revision October 2003, APHIS, USDA, Harvard Center for Risk Assessment (www.hcra.harvard.edu).

"FDA Asked to Rescind Use of Carbon Monoxide for Meats," *FoodNavigator.com*, November 17, 2005.

"FDA Issues Guidance on GMO Safety Testing," *FoodNavigator.com*, June 23, 2006.

"FDA Proposes Consumer Study on Food Labels Carb Claims," *Food Label News* (www.foodlabels.com), 6, no. 5, (2005).

"FDA Warns Milk Producers to Remove 'Hormone Free' Claims from the Labeling of Dairy Products," FDA News, Washington, D.C., September 12, 2003.

Federoff, Nina, Ph.D., and Nancy Marie Brown. *Mendel in the Kitchen: A Scientist's View of Genetically Modified Foods*. Washington, D.C.: Joseph Henry Press, 2004.

"Final Organic Rules," *Federal Register*, 65, no. 246 (2000): 80668.

"Flame Retardants Found in U.S. Food Test," MSNBC.com, September 1, 2004.

"Food Irradiation: A Safe Measure," *FDA Consumer* magazine, January 2000.

Foran, Jeffery A. "Dioxin-Contaminated Farmed Salmon: Foren et al. Respond," *Environmental Health Perspectives*, correspondence, 113, no. 14 (2005).

Forgrieve, Janet. "Painful Spurt for Organic Foods," *Rocky Mountain News*, July 8, 2006.

Fromartz, Samuel. *Organic Inc.: Natural Foods and How They Grew* (Chapter 4: "A Spring Mix"; Chapter 5: "Mythic Manufacturing"; Chapter 6: "Backlash"). New York: Harcourt, 2006.

Gaik, Ong Beng (Consumer's Association of Penang). "Misuse and Overuse of Antibiotics: Who Is to Blame," TWN Third World Network (www.twnside .org.sg).

"GM Crop Watch: FAO Calls for All-Round Control," *FoodNavigator.com*, January 1, 2005.

"GM Dispute Panel Meets in Geneva," *FoodNavigator.com*, February 18, 2005.

"GM Pea Study Discontinued After Assessment Failure," *FoodNavigator.com*, November 21, 2005.

Gogoi, Pallavi. "Wal-Mart's Organic Offensive," *BusinessWeek Online*, March 29, 2006.

Heller, Lorraine. "Horizon Dairy Targeted for Lacking Organic Practices," *Dairy Reporter*, August 8, 2006.

————. "Labeling Seminar Outline Anticipated FDA Changes," *FoodNavigator.com*, June 23, 2006.

Hellmich, Nancy. "Atkins: Have We Had Our Fill?" *USA Today*, August 1, 2005.

———— and Steve Sternberg, "Atkins Wasn't Obese, Hospital File Shows," *USA Today*, February 10, 2004.

Hites, Ronald A., Jeffery A. Foran, et al. "Global Assessment of Organic Contaminants in Farmed Salmon," *Science*, 303, January 9, 2004.

Hou, Z., S. Sang, et al. "Mechanism of Action of EGCG Auto-oxidation-dependent Inactivation of Epidermal Growth Factor Receptor and Direct Effects on Growth Inhibition in Human Esophageal Cancer KYSE Cells," *Cancer Research*, 65, no. 17 (2005).

"The Incredible Inedible Egg," *Chicago Tribune*, June 15, 2001.

"Japan Ends Blanket BSE Test Rule," *Food & Drink Weekly*, May 16, 2005.

Jensen, Helen H., and Dermot J. Hayes. "Antibiotics Restrictions: Taking Stock of Denmark's Experience," *Iowa Ag Review*, 9, no. 3 (2003).

Jin, Y., C. H. Jin, et al. "Separation of Catechin Compounds from Different Teas," *Biotechnology Journal*, 1, no. 2 (2006).

Kane, Linda. "A Recipe for Scampi: How It Really Gets to Your Table," *Customs and Border Protections Today*, December 2004.

Karnowski, Steven. "Organic Family Dairy Operations Wary as Corporations Move In," Associated Press, *Lansing State Journal*, June 30, 2006.

Kastel, Mark Alan. "Maintaining the Integrity of Organic Milk, Showcasing Ethical Family Farm Producers, Exposing the Corporate Takeover—Factory Farm Production," Cornucopia Institute, Cornucopia, Wisconsin, April 19, 2006.

Kelleher, Colm, Ph.D. *Brain Trust*. New York: Paraview, 2004.

Kilman, Scott. "Tyson Foods to Curb Use of Baytril," *The Wall Street Journal*, February 20, 2002.

Kim, W., M. H. Jeong, et al. "Effect of Green Tea Consumption on Endothelial Function and Circulating Endothelial Progenitor Cells in Chronic Smokers," *Circulation*, 70, no. 8 (2006).

Kuma, K., S. C. Gupta, et al. "Antibiotic Uptake by Plants from Soil Fertilization with Animal Manure," *Journal of Environmental Quality*, 34 (2005).

Kurtzweil, Paula. "Skimming the Milk Label: Fat Reduced Milk Products Join the Food Labeling Fold, *FDA Consumer* magazine, January 1, 1998.

"Labeling and Children Key If Food Industry to Avoid Legislation," *FoodNavigator.com*, April, 1, 2005.

"Label Properly or Lose Consumer Trust, Warns NHB," *FoodNavigator.com*, June 10, 2005.

Lavigne, Paula. "Is Organic the Real Deal?" *The Dallas Morning News*, July 17, 2006.

Leeds, Margot Roosevelt. "Got Hormones: The Simmering Issue of Milk Labels Boils Over When an Agrochemical Giant Sues Small Farmers in Maine," *Time* magazine, December 22, 2003.

Lim, V. K., Y. M. Cheong, and A. B. Suleiman. "Pattern of Antibiotic Usage in Hospitals in Malaysia," *Singapore Medical Journal*, 34, no. 6 (1993).

"Low Carb Craze," *News Hour with Jim Lehrer*, National Public Radio, April 23, 2004 (transcript at www.pbs.org).

May, Thomas. "Organic Food Trends for the Year Ahead," *The Natural Foods Merchandiser*, January 1, 2003.

Mazdai, Anita, Nathan Dodder, et al. "Polybrominated Diphenyl Ethers in Maternal and Fetal Blood Samples," *Environmental Health Perspectives*, 111, no. 9 (2003).

McCaig, Linda F., M.P.H., Richard Besser, M.D., and James M. Hughes, M.D. "Trends in Antimicrobial Prescribing Rates for Children and Adolescents," *The Journal of the American Medical Association (JAMA)*, 287, no. 23 (2002).

Mellon, Margaret, Ph.D. "Hogging It! Estimates of Antimicrobial Abuse in Livestock," Union of Concerned Scientists (www.ucsusa.org), January 2001.

Mergentime, Ken, and Monica Emerich, "Organic Fraud Case Deepens: Possible Link Causes OCIA Turmoil," *The Natural Foods Merchandiser*, March 1995.

Middaugh, John P., Scott M. Arnold, and Lori Verbrugge. "Risk Based Consumption of Dioxin-Contaminated Farmed Salmon," *Environmental Health Perspectives*, correspondence, 113, no. 14 (2005).

Molbak, K. "Spread of Resistant Bacteria and Resistant Genes from Animals to Humans—The Public Health Consequences," *Journal of Veterinary Medicine*, 51, no. 8–9 (2004).

Mozaffarian, Dariush, M.D., Martijn B. Katan, et al. "Trans Fatty Acids and Cardiovascular Disease," *New England Journal of Medicine*, 354, no. 15 (2006).

Nagle, D. G., D. Ferreira, et al. "Epigallocatechin-3-gallate (EGCG): Chemical and Biomedical Perspectives," *Phytochemistry*, July 28, 2006.

Navarro, Luis Hernandez."To Die a Little: Migration and Coffee in Mexico and Central America," Americas Program at the Interhemispheric Resource Center (americas.irc-online.org), December 13, 2004.

Naylor, Rosamond L. "Environmental Safeguards for Open-Ocean Aquaculture," *Issues in Science and Technology*, spring of 2006.

"New Dietary Guidelines Promote Heart Health," *FoodNavigator.com*, June 21, 2006.

"Nine Arrested for Fake Virgin Olive Oil Fraud," *Expatica*, Barcelona, Spain, April 12, 2006.

Norton, Amy. "The Corn Next Door: Can Organic and Biotech Crops Coexist?" *The Scientist*, 19, no. 18 (2005).

"Omega-3s now in Bacon and Pork Chops: Omega-3 Pork Without Genetic Modification," *Supermarket Guru* (www.supermarketguru.com), March 28 and April 4, 2006.

"Optics Tackle Olive Oil Fraud," IOP Publishing Limited, Optics.org, November 28, 2003.

"Organic Food Fraud Sends Shockwaves Through Sector," *FoodNavigator.com*, May 18, 2006.

Organic Foods Production Act of 1990, National Organic Program, USDA.

Otto, Daniel, Ph.D., and Theresa Varner. "Consumers, Vendors, and the Economic Importance of Iowa Farmers' Markets: An Economic Impact Survey Analysis," Iowa State University, March 2005.

"Pacific White Shrimp: U.S. Demand Just Keeps on Growing, As Does Global Production Despite Economic and Natural Setbacks," *SeaFood Business*, July 2006.

"Palm Oil 'Reasonable' Replacement for Trans Fats, Say Experts," *FoodNavigator.com*, December 16, 2005.

Paulson, Steven. "Awash in Loss: N.E. Colorado Farmers Fear a Court Ruling Will Cost Them Their Livelihood and Land as Well as Their Water," *The Denver Post*, July 10, 2006.

"PDO: The Great Hope for Cheese Makers?" *FoodNavigator.com*, April 29, 2003.

"Perdue to Stop Using Antibiotics," Associated Press, February 28, 2002.

"Pesticide Data Program" annual summary calendar for year 2003, Agricultural Marketing Service (AMS), USDA.

Pollack, Andrew. "No Altered Corn Found in Allergy Samples," The New York Times, July 11, 2001.

Price, Lance B., Elizabeth Johnson, et al. "Floroquinolone-Resistant Campylobacter Isolates from Conventional and Antibiotic Free Chicken Products," Environmental Health Perspectives, 113, no. 5 (2005).

Quaid, Libby. "U.S. Plans to Scale Back Testing for Mad Cow Disease," Associated Press, The Wall Street Journal, March 14, 2006.

Raabe, Steve. "Organic Farm Under Fire Over Pasture Rules," The Denver Post, January 16, 2005.

"Rapid Test to Detect E. Coli Bacteria," FoodNavigator.com, March 19, 2002.

Ready, Ben. "Dairy Debate: USDA Investigation into Local Company Puts Spotlight in Fight Over Organic Labeling," The Daily Times-Call, Longmont, Colorado, April, 10, 2006.

"Riding the Higher Range: The Story of Colorado's Coleman Ranch and Coleman Natural Beef," published by Glen Melvin Coleman, Boulder, Colorado: Johnson Printing, 1998.

"Risks and Benefits of Eating Fish Debated," Harvard Public Health NOW, March 3, 2006.

Ruiz-Marrero, Carmelo. "Clouds on Organic Horizon: Is Organic Farming Becoming the Victim of Its Own Success?" CorpWatch (www.corpwatch.org), November 25, 2004.

Ruland, Susan. "Milk's Safety" (letter to the editor), Chicago Tribune, June 13, 2006.

Ruttenberg, Jim. "Media Talk: Report on Organic Foods Is Challenged," The New York Times, July 31, 2000.

"Safe Food Handling," "Meat Packaging Materials," fact sheets, Food Safety and Inspection Service, USDA.

Samuels, Adrienne P. "Record Showers Bring June Glowers," The Boston Globe, June 26, 2006.

Schecter, Arnold, Marian Pavuk, et al. "Polybrominated Diphenyl Ethers (PBDEs) in U.S. Mothers' Milk," Environmental Health Perspectives, 111, no. 14 (2003).

Scott, Mary. "Olive Oil Company Accused of Fraud," The Natural Foods Merchandiser, December 1997.

"Seafood Companies, Individual Plead Guilty to Fish Fraud," Associated Press, August 11, 2006.

Severson, Kim. "An Organic Cash Cow," The New York Times, November 9, 2005.

———— and Cindy Burke. *The Trans Fat Solution*, Berkeley, California: Ten Speed Press, 2003.

Shaneyfelt, Terrence, Rozita Husein, Glenn Bubley, and Christos S. Mantzoros. "Hormonal Predictors of Prostate Cancer: A Meta-Analysis," *Journal of Clinical Oncology*, 18, no. 4 (2000).

Shapin, Stephen. "Paradise Sold: What Are You Buying When You Buy Organic?" *The New Yorker*, May 15, 2006.

"Smart Label Senses Quality of Package Meat," *FoodNavigator.com*, July 3, 2006.

Steele, Jeremy. "Farmers See Growth in More Natural Crops," *Lansing State Journal*, July 10, 2006.

Steinman, G. "Mechanisms of Twinning, VII: Effect of the Diet and Heredity on the Human Twinning Rate," *The Journal of Reproductive Medicine*, 51, no. 5 (2006).

Stewart, Kimberly Lord. "Fresh, Natural and . . . Confusing," *The Denver Post*, August 6, 2003.

————. "Meat-Label Madness," *The Natural Foods Merchandiser*, March 2003.

————. "Olive Oil's Slippery Supply Line: Italian Extra-Virgin not Always Real Thing," *The Denver Post*, October 26, 2003.

————. "Virtuosity: Is the Olive-Oil Industry Fraught with Fraud?" *Better Nutrition*, February 2003.

"Supermarket Chains Refuse to Sell Carbon Monoxide–Treated Meat," ConsumerAffairs.com, April 6, 2006.

"Top Poultry Processors Faulted for High Salmonella Rates," *FoodNavigator.com*, July, 7, 2006.

"The Use of Drugs in Food Animals: Benefits and Risks, Panel on Animal Health, Food Safety, and Public Health," National Research Council, Washington, D.C., 2004.

"U.S. Food Giants Attacked Over 'Low Sugar' Claims," *FoodNavigator.com*, February 30, 2005.

"U.S. Per Capita Food Consumption," Economic Research Service, USDA, December ?1, 2005.

"U.S. Survey Reveals Most Americans Unaware of Antibiotics in Meat," *Food Production Daily*, May 5, 2003.

Waldman, Peter. "Levels of Risk: Common Industrial Chemicals in Tiny Doses Raise Health Issue," *The Wall Street Journal*, July 25, 2005.

Wallace, Sarah. "Feds Seize Gallons of Impure Olive Oil in Bust," WABC News (New York), February 9, 2006.

Wambach, Jessica. "Bacterial Illness Linked to Raw Milk Infecting More People," *Yakima Herald-Republic* (Yakima, Washington), March 30, 2006.

Wargo, John. *Our Children's Toxic Legacy* (Chapter 9: "The Diet of a Child"). New Haven, CT: Yale University Press, 1998.

Warner, Melanie. "Wal-Mart Eyes Organic Foods," *The New York Times,* May 12, 2006.

Weise, Elizabeth. "BBB: 'Animal Care Certified' Isn't All It's Cracked Up to Be: Complaint Charges Egg Logo Overstates Humane Care of Hens," *USA Today,* August 29, 2004.

———. "Cage Free Hens Pushed to Rule the Roost," *USA Today,* May 10, 2006.

Weiss, Kenneth R. "Struggling Sea Lions: Marine Mammals Under Attack by Ocean Toxins," *Los Angeles Times,* September 4, 2006.

Wheeler, Larry. "Snapper Standoff: Some Say Restrictions Needed; Others Fearful," *Pensacola News Journal,* August 30, 2006.

Whittaker, Debbie. "Colorado Quinoa: Transplanted from the Andes," Front Range Living (www.frontrangeliving.com), August 2006.

Wieberg, Theresa. "Fishy Debate: Groups Argue Over Salmon's Benefit to Pregnant Moms," ABCNews.com, February 23, 2006.

Worthington, Virginia, M.S., Sc.D., C.N.S. "Effect of Agricultural Methods on Nutritional Quality: A Comparison of Organic and Conventional Crops," *Alternative Therapies,* 4 (1998): 58–69.

Yoon, Carol Kaesuk. "Altered Corn May Imperil Butterfly, Researchers Say," *The New York Times,* May 20, 1999.

Zehner, David. "An Economic Assessment of Fair Trade in Coffee," *Chazen Web Journal of International Business,* Columbia Business School, Columbia University School of International and Public Affairs, fall 2002.

During the writing of this book, the author interviewed the following people: Mark and May Belle Adams, residents, Neosho, Missouri; Dr. Khosrow Adeli, Head and Professor of Clinical Biochemistry, the Hospital for Sick Children, University of Toronto; Alex Avery, Director of Research and Education, Center for Global Food Issues; Deanna Baldwin, Maryland Department of Agriculture, College of Agricultural Science, Penn State, and board member, National Egg Regulatory Officials (NERO); Neil Blomquist, former CEO and president, Spectrum Naturals; Haven Bourque, TransFair USA; Mel Coleman, Jr., Chairman, Coleman Natural Meats; Katherine DiMatteo, former Executive Director, Organic Trade Association; Clark Driftmier, Senior Vice President of Marketing, Aurora Organic Dairy; Rex Dufour, agricultural specialist, National Sustainable Agricultural Information Service (NCAT, ATTRA); Roberta Larson Dyuff, Canned Food Alliance; Tom German, owner, Thankful Harvest; Tom Green, Board of Directors, IPM

Institute of North America, and President, IPMWorks; Peter Holt, PhD., microbiologist, Egg Safety and Quality, USDA; Stephen L. Joseph, founder, president, and legal representative, BanTransFats.com, Inc.; Thor Lassen, president, Ocean Trust; Richard Lobb, Director of Communications, National Chicken Board; David Lynch, owner, Guidestone Farm; William Marler, Seattle trial attorney; Antonio Marulli and Catherine Amey, Monte della Torre, Sparanese, Italy; Gale Mason, Assistant National Supervisor, Shell Eggs, Grading Branch, USDA; Margaret Mellon, Ph.D., Director of the Food and Environment Program, Union of Concerned Scientists; William More, vice president, Aquaculture Certification Council; Jo Natale, Director of Media Relations, Wegmans; Rodney North, Equal Exchange, Inc.; Eli Saddler, Public Health Analyst, Got Mercury?; Kathy Seuss, Farm Program and Public Education Manager, Food Animal Concern Trust (FACT); Paul Shapiro, Campaign Director, COK; Dennis Stiffler, Ph.D., Executive Vice President of Food Safety, Coleman Natural Meats; Diane Storey, spokesperson, United Egg Producers, and account supervisor, Golin Harris; Cyd Szymanski, Nest Fresh Eggs; Jule Taylor, vice president, Milk Supply, Horizon Organic Dairy; Dave Turunjian, Hillside Egg Farm; Liz Wagstrom, D.V.M., Assistant Vice President of Science and Technology, National Pork Board; Stacey Zawel, Ph.D., Beans for Health Alliance.

(continued from page iv)
New Hampshire; Sample Nutrition Facts courtesy of Center for Food Safety and Applied Nutrition, FDA; Seafood Safe logo courtesy of Eco Fish, Dover, New Hampshire, www.ecofish.com; Smart Choices logo courtesy of PepsiCo, Purchase, New York, www.pepsico.com; Stamp of the 1906 Pure Food and Drugs Act by artist Carl Herrman courtesy of the United States Postal Service, Washington, D.C.; Tested Quality logo courtesy of Pennsylvania Egg Quality Assurance Program (PEQAP), Pennsylvania Department of Agriculture, Harrisburg, Pennsylvania, www.agriculture.state.pa.us; United Egg Producers Certified symbol courtesy of United Egg Producers; USDA Organic, Prime, Choice, Select, A Grade, AA Grade, Inspected for Wholesomeness Department of Agriculture, and MyPyramid.gov symbols courtesy of USDA; Whole Grains logos courtesy of Whole Grains Council, Boston, Massachusetts, www.wholegrainscouncil.org.